MW01528885

CBD Hemp Oil.
A users guide

By

Robert McGowan

Contents

@Copyright 2018 by Robert McGowan - All rights reserved.

The following eBook is reproduced with the goal of providing information that is as accurate and reliable as possible. The recommendations suggestions contained in these pages are solely for entertainment purposes. Before undertaking any action based on the contents of this book, consult a medical health professional.

This declaration is deemed fair and valid by both the American Bar Association and the Committee of Publishers Association and is legally binding throughout the United States.

Furthermore, the transmission, duplication or reproduction of any of the following work in any form (including specific information) is illegal. This extends to creating a secondary or tertiary copy of the work. No record copy of this work can me produced without with the express, written consent from the publisher. All additional rights reserved.

The information in the following pages is broadly considered to be a truthful and accurate account of facts and, as such, any inattention, use or misuse of the information in question by the reader will render any resulting actions solely under his/her purview. There are no instances in which the publisher or the original author of this work can be deemed liable for any hardship or damages that may befall them after undertaking information described herein.

Additionally, the information in the following pages is intended only for informational purposes and should thus be regarded as universal. As befitting its nature, it is presented without assurance regarding its prolonged validity or interim quality. Trademarks that are mentioned are done without written consent and can in no way be considered an endorsement from the trademark holder.

6

Dedication

For my mum and dad.

Thank you for giving me the strength to reach for the stars and chase my dreams.

I love you both.

-   Robert

Introduction

It is mysterious and unknown. It has saved lives. Though still illegal in many parts of our world, many people say it is a miracle. The reality is that CBD oil can relieve anxiety, diminish or eliminate seizures, and alleviate pain.

The power of CBD oil continues to grow. From social media advertisements to informational videos, increasing numbers of people are heralding the wonders of natural cannabinoids, hoping to increase the groundswell to make marijuana legal. Men and women continue to celebrate the successes they have encountered from CBD oil. And we want to share their joy with you.

The battle against marijuana continues to rage. Because of the legal classification of marijuana and CBD, many people are afraid to try them. But, they are missing out. While the government may not have caught up, countless people have started using CBD oil – and their health is better than ever.

This book will address CBD oil and its uses. CBD oil's applications continue to expand – it is a wonder!

In the following pages, you will learn about the amazing benefits of this oil, where it came from, what differentiates it from marijuana, the best ways to pick out the right type of oil, and how to use it. When you finish this quick and easy read, you will be better prepared to use CBD oil to your health's benefit.

Thank you for buying this book. If you enjoy reading it, please leave a review on Amazon!

Chapter 1: The History of Cannabis

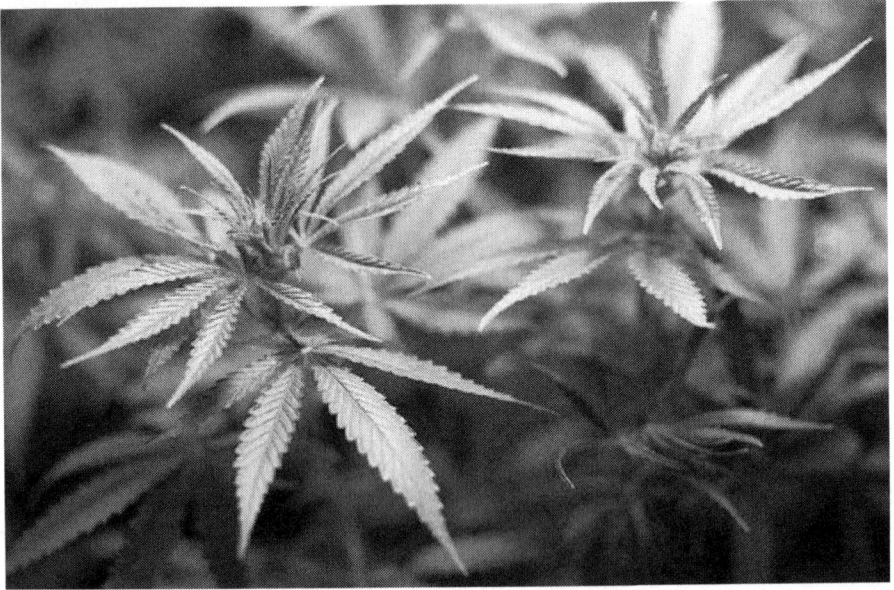

The history of cannabis is long and shows how this plant has been around in many different countries much longer than we may have originally realized. A report by Barney Warf describes how cannabis use originated in Asia thousands of years ago before it slowly moved to other regions of the world, and eventually came to the United States and the Americas.

In the beginning, cannabis was used for spiritual and medicinal purposes. People did not use it to get high or for some of the other uses that are so popular today. Instead, those who were looking for a spiritual journey or who were performing spiritual rituals would use the cannabis to help enhance the experience. There are many societies that have been able to use cannabis and the different parts of the plant as a form of medicine to treat a variety of illnesses. For example, the medieval Germans and the Vikings were known to use cannabis to help relieve the pain associated with toothaches and childbirth. Industrial Hemp was grown and spun into usable fibers and textiles.

The idea that cannabis is an evil thing, like what we hear about in our modern media, is relatively recent. And the fact that the United States sees marijuana as an illegal substance runs counter to the plant's history.

Where did cannabis come from?

It is important to recognize that there are two familiar subspecies of the cannabis plant. First, *Cannabis sativa*, known as marijuana, is the part with psychoactive properties. The second part, known as *Cannabis sativa L.*, is the subspecies known as hemp and it does not have any psychoactive properties. This is the type that is going to be used for making a variety of products such as fuel, cloth, and oil.

There is also a second species of the cannabis plant that is also psychoactive, known as *Cannabis indica*, which was identified by Jean-Baptiste Lamarck, as well as a third one, which is pretty uncommon, known as *Cannabis rederalis,* named by the Russian botanist D.E. Janischevisky.

Cannabis plants are believed to be evolved from Central Asia. It is believed that they were found mostly in the regions we now know as southern Siberia and Mongolia. The history of cannabis can be traced back 12,000 years, placing it amongst humanity's oldest cultivated crops.

Cannabis did well in this particular area of Asia because it was found in areas that were full of nutrients from dump sites of hunters and gatherers. Burned cannabis seeds have also been found in the burial mounds of Siberia as far back as 3000 B.C. and

11

in nobles from the Xinjian region of Siberia and China as far back as 2500 B.C.

Both psychoactive marijuana and hemp were believed to be widely used in ancient China, which makes sense considering the remnants found in so many areas of the country. The first record of the drug being used for a medicinal purpose is dated around 4000 B.C. One of the ways cannabis was used for ancient medicine was as a type of anesthetic during surgery. It is believed that the Chinese Emperor Shen Nung used cannabis for this purpose in 2737 B.C.

So, how did cannabis spread out from China to other parts of the world? Coastal farmers started to bring pot to Korea in 2000 B.C., although there are some researchers who believe it may have happened before this time. Cannabis started to move to the South Asian subcontinent sometime between 2000 B.C. and 1000 B.C. when the region was invaded by the Aryans, a group that was able to speak in an archaic Indo-European Language.

The cannabis drug continued to spread as more of the world's populations began to mix together, either through trade or war. The drug quickly caught on in India, where it was celebrated as one of the five kingdoms of herbs that were able to release the user from anxiety. In fact, in the poem "Science of Charms" the powers of cannabis were heralded for all to hear.

How cannabis moved from Asia to Europe

Cannabis slowly started to move away from China and into other parts of the world. It is believed that it showed up in the Middle East sometime between 2000 and 1400 B.C. and it was used there by a group known as the Scythians. The Scythians likely carried the drug into other areas, including Ukraine and southeast Russia, since they are known to have occupied the territories for many years.

From there, Germanic tribes took the drug into their homeland. When the invasion of Britain took place in the 5th century, cannabis went with the soldiers.

Remnants of cannabis seeds have been found in the remains of many Viking ships dated to the mid-ninth century.

Over the following centuries, cannabis slowly started to migrate to the different regions of the world. It went not only through Europe and the different parts of Asia, but also started to travel through Africa. It reached South American in the 19th century and over time, and as more people started to travel, eventually made its way over to the Americas, including North America.

When did cannabis get to the United States?

It took a while before cannabis came to the United States. It is believed the plant finally made its way over here during the 20th century, arriving from Mexico to the southwest part of the country when immigrants fled during the Mexican Revolution.

It is believed that some of the early prejudices against cannabis and the way that it was used were racist fears against the people who used it. It was not uncommon for local newspapers to blame Mexicans for smoking marijuana, for property crimes, for going on murder sprees, and for seducing children.

Most of the laws in America never recognized the difference between *Cannabis sativa* and *Cannabis sativa L*. The plant was first outlawed in Utah in 1915 and by 1931, 29 states had made it plant illegal regardless of the specific form. Even if people wanted to use the non-psychoactive form of the drug, this is illegal in most states in the United States.

In 1930, Harry Aslinger, the first commissioner of the FBN (Federal Bureau of Narcotics) worked to make marijuana illegal throughout the whole country. In 1937, the Marijuana Tax Act moved the regulation of cannabis to the Drug Enforcement Agency, basically criminalizing both possession and use in all parts of the country.

This has made it hard for many to possess cannabis. Even if you use it as a medicine, or in a religious ceremony, the drug is considered illegal. While a few states have started to legalize cannabis, it is still seen as an illegal substance, regardless of the use.

Today, the federal government classifies marijuana as a Schedule I controlled substance along with LSD and heroin. The main reason deals with fear that the psychoactive option of the plant will lead to addiction and abuse. The government does not look at the accepted medical uses nor does it recognize that there could be a safe level of use.

Many people in the United States have started to protest repressive cannabis laws. Some states have succeeded in making the plant legal. However, even if the cannabis is allowed in the state where you live, you still have to be careful about use and you cannot possess it in states where it is illegal – even if you purchased legally in another state.

Studies on cannabis

While this book will talk about cannabis and some of the good effects it can have on the body, it is important to realize that there are limited studies. Cannabis, despite all its benefits, is still illegal in most of the United States and most of the western world including the U.K.

Because cannabis is illegal in most parts of the western world, it is hard to conduct studies on its effects and benefits. The studies we have are limited to a few patients who have been able to get help from a doctor to take the cannabis or those who live in areas where cannabis is legal.

As more areas in the United States and the United Kingdom start to abolish the laws that make cannabis illegal, there will be more studies on how cannabis works and even more about the benefits you can receive by taking cannabis. The good news is that the available studies are very promising regarding how good cannabis, especially CBD, can be for your overall health.

Chapter 2: What is CBD Oil?

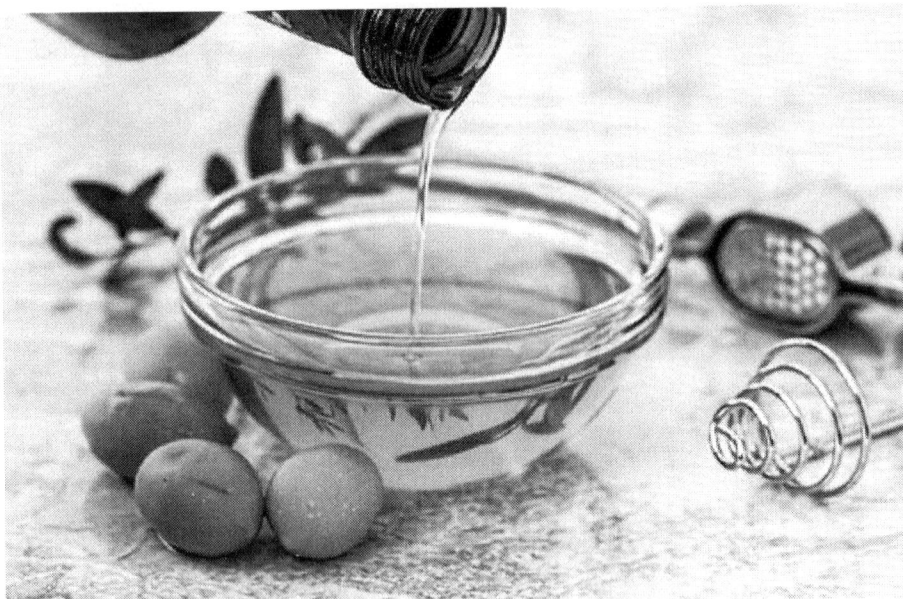

Even though many countries and regions of the world have been using cannabis and the different parts of its plant for centuries as a spiritual tool and for medicinal purposes, many modern countries have seen it as a bad thing and made the plant illegal until recently. And since cannabis has slowly seen itself become legal again, the world, and the scientific community just can't seem to get enough of this plant.

While those who are against the legalization of cannabis worry that those who want access to cannabis are just looking to get high, most people actually aren't after this at all. Rather, they are interested in the cannabis plant because of the great medicine it can provide. One of the best and most potent ways to get all of the good that comes with the cannabis plant without any of the unwanted effects comes from using either CBD hemp oil or CBD cannabis oil.

What is CBD Oil?

CBD oil, or cannabidiol oil, is made from strains of the cannabis plant with low levels of **tetrahydrocannabinol** (THC). THC is the part of the cannabis plant that makes marijuana psychoactive and will give you a high. Rather than containing THC, CBD oil is high in cannabinoids, which is a group of phytochemicals found inside the cannabis plant in a natural and safe form.

Cannabis has been used throughout the world for a long time to treat illnesses and diseases. This history has been stifled a bit in the Western world due to the fact that cannabis in all forms has been seen as illegal. But as the legal status of cannabis starts to change, the stigma is lifting as well, and more people are looking to this treatment to improve their health.

Cannabinoids are healthy and good for your body. In fact, there are many plants already in use to promote health that contain these substances in a natural form. In addition, the human body creates its own cannabinoids and it has millions of receptors for this substance, found mainly in the immune system, central nervous system, and the brain.

Cannabinoids already play a huge role in the body. The endocannabinoid system regulates homeostasis, or a general state of balance in the body. Subsequently, this substance can impact different parts of the body such as your response to pain, your immune response, hormone regulation, appetite, sleep, and even your mood. Only recently has science been able to take a closer look at cannabinoids than their effects on human health, which means that we have just scratched the surface on all the cool things CBD oil can do for you.

Until recently, the best-known compound from the cannabis plant was THC because it is the most active ingredient found in marijuana. Marijuana actually contains both CBD and THC, but these compounds are found in different amounts in marijuana and they are going to have different effects.

THC is so well-known because it has the ability to make the user feel high by influencing the way the mind works. This happens whenever THC is broken down with the use of heat and then introduced into the body, such as when you cook it into foods or smoke the plant.

While THC is known to be psychoactive, CBD is not. This means that while you are able to get some great changes to the body and enjoy some medical benefits from using CBD, it does not change the state of the user's mind. Most of the time, if CBD is going to be used in a medicinal manner, it is found in the least processed form of the plant, which is called hemp. Hemp and marijuana both come from the same plant, *Cannabis sativa*, but they are very different.

Hemp farmers do not modify the plant because they want it to stay as natural as possible for medicinal purposes. Hemp plants are used to produce the CBD used on many common ailments.

How CBD oil works

All cannabinoids work by attaching themselves to receptors inside the body to produce their effects. It is natural for the body itself to produce some cannabinoids on its own. The human body has two main receptors for cannabinoids known as the CB1 and CB2 receptors.

The CB1 receptors are found all over the body, which means you could use these cannabinoids everywhere. However, most of these receptors are found in the brain. The CB1 receptors in the brain deal with all kinds of movement and coordination along with memories, appetite, thinking, mood and emotions, and even pain. THC attaches specifically to these receptors. Effects can generally take from 20 minutes to up to three hours – the time often depends on the amount consumed and the method of consumption.

On the other hand, the CB2 receptors are more commonly found in the immune system. They work to reduce pain and inflammation in the body.

The thoughts surrounding CBD oil have changed. It was once believed that CBD acted with the CB2 receptors. However, it now seems that CBD oil does not really react with either receptor in a direct manner. Instead, it works to influence the body to use more of its own natural cannabinoids to get things done.

The Uses of CBD Oil

While we will go into this a bit more later on, it is important to note all of the great uses for CBD oil. Remember this is all natural and allows you to enjoy the healing benefits from this plant, without any of the unwanted effects. People have used cannabis for its medicinal purposes for years, and CBD allows you to do this without causing any harm to the body.

There are a lot of uses for CBD oil, especially if you get a high-quality product. From a healing perspective, CBD oil can treat symptoms of:

- ADHD
- Anxiety
- Autism
- Cancer
- Seizures
- Pain

- Headaches
- Pain during childbirth
- And much more

Below are some examples of how to use CBD.

Help increase appetite in cancer patients: 2.5 milligrams of THC by mouth with or without 1 mg of CBD for six weeks.
For chronic pain: 2.5-20 mg CBD by mouth for an average of 25 days.
Help manage epilepsy: 200-300 mg of CBD by mouth daily.
Help with movement problems associated with Huntington's disease: 10 mg per kilogram of CBD by mouth daily for six weeks.
Treat sleeping disorders: 40-160 mg CBD by mouth.
Manage multiple sclerosis symptoms: Cannabis plant extracts containing 2.5-120 milligrams of a THC-CBD combination by mouth daily for 2-15 weeks. A mouth spray might contain 2.7 milligrams of THC and 2.5 milligrams of CBD at doses of 2.5-120 milligram for up to eight weeks. Patients typically use eight sprays within any three hours, with a maximum of 48 sprays in any 24-hour period.
Help treat schizophrenia: 40-1,280 mg CBD by mouth daily.
Treat glaucoma: a single CBD dose of 20-40 mg under the tongue. Doses greater than 40 mg could potentially increase eye pressure.

As you can see, many people can benefit from using CBD oil to make themselves healthier. There is a changing tide and an ever-growing group of people who are certain that the cannabis plant is good for them and that prohibitory laws need to be overturned. As more information comes out about cannabis and the good it can do for people, especially the form that does not have any THC the more likely that the illegal status of cannabis will be overturned, benefitting everyone.

The different strains of CBD

There are quite a few different strains of CBD based on how strong they are, how much CBD is inside of them, and even how much THC. Each one will work a bit differently on your symptoms based on the chemicals it contains. Let's take a look at some of the top strains of CBD to show the differences.

Charlotte's Web

Charlotte's Web is a good option for those who are looking to treat seizures. It has 0.3% THC in it, so the medical potency comes from the high-CBD content. The Stanley Brothers specifically cultivated this strain to help epileptic patients. It has since grown in popularity as a great hemp-based medication that allows patients to perform regular daily tasks. For some patients, it is common to feel dizziness when you first start taking Charlotte's Web, so use with caution.

Harlequin

Harlequin is another option when you are looking for strains of CBD. This is a 75/25 sativa-dominant strain best known because of its reliable expression of CBD. It is a descendant of a few different types of CBD including Nepali indica, Colombian Gold, Thai, and Swiss Landrace. Because it has a 5:2 ratio of CBD to THC, this strain is the best for treating anxiety and pain. Many people also choose this option because there are different flavorings, which makes it easier to consume. If you are looking for a way to relax and deal with pain without being sedated, Harlequin is the best option for you.

Sour Tsunami

Sour Tsunami is a strain known as the very first with a CBD content that is higher than its THC content. The result is that Sour Tsunami is good at treating inflammation and pain without producing unwanted side effects. CBD levels in this are up to 10 percent. It is a cross between NYC Diesel and Sour Diesel and it comes with a musky, diesel smell with some sweet undertones.

Cannatonic

This strain is a unique hybrid from Spain that has a THC content below six percent and a high CBD content that can be above 17 percent. It is a cross between the female MK Ultra and the male G13 Haze; it is used to help relax and mellow you out. It is considered one of the premier medical strains, so it will treat migraines, anxiety, muscle spasms, and pain.

Colombian Gold

This is a classic, landrace sativa that started in the Santa Marta mountains of Colombia. The buds are fluffy and crystal-covered with some sweet scents. This is a good strain to go with to help reduce anxiety. It can help you to stay productive at the same time. It is also used for many physical symptoms like pain and muscle tension. It stimulates users and helps them feel happier as well, which is why Colombian Gold can be used to treat ADD/ADHD and depression.

Sour Diesel

This strain is sometimes known as "Sour D" and it is an invigorating strain of CBD. It works fast and can help to energize the brain in no time, making it the perfect option to deal with depression, pain, and stress. It also lasts for a long time, making it a top choice for many medical patients.

MK Ultra

This is the strain to use for some really powerful cerebral affects. It is a cross between G-13 and OG Kush and it was bred by T.H. Seeds. It is best known for giving the patient an almost hypnotic effect and it works fast. It is a good, strong medication when needed. It is a bit stronger than the other strains, so it is best to take only on days when you are able to relax and let its effects work.

Super Skunk

This is predominantly an *indica* variety that comes from its parent strain known as "Skunk #1." This strain is good for producing a bold and relaxing effect all over the body. Patients who use this strain find that it helps them deal with many aches and pains of the body and can reduce stress levels.

G13

G13 is a strong strain of *Cannabis indica* that has many urban legends around it. Some accounts say that the FBI and CIA gathered the best marijuana strains in the world and then used those to grow new hybrids. Then, an unnamed technician released it to the masses – G13. Although it is unlikely that these stories are true, G13 delivers effects like nothing else and can be great for medicinal uses.

Each of these strains offers something unique to the customer and it often depends on what you are trying to treat and how strong you need the relief to be. Researching each of these options more can help ensure that you get the best strain for your needs.

Chapter 3: How CBD Oil Works on the Body and Mind – The Short-Medium-Long Term Effects

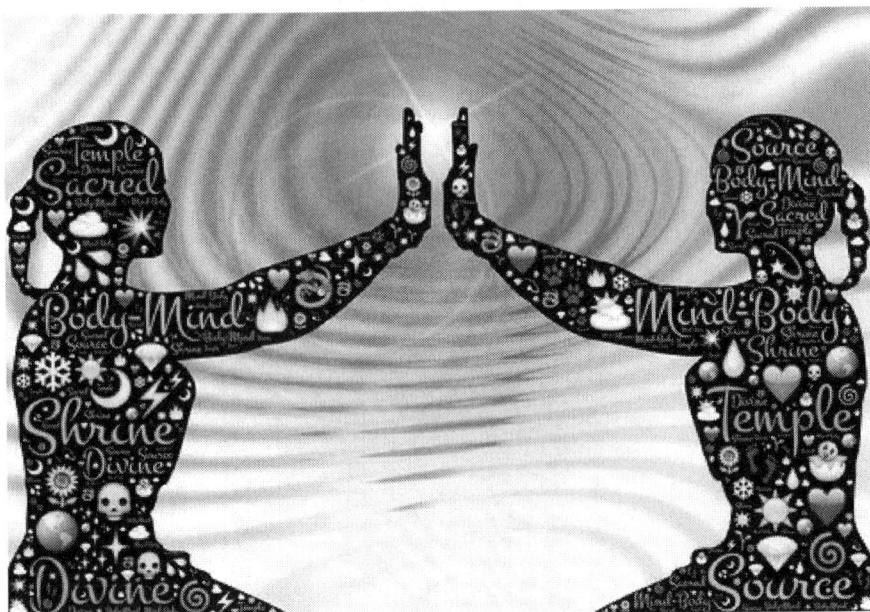

While cannabis and the different parts of the plant have spent many years being seen as evil by those in the commercial as well as scientific world, they are starting to get a new name. More people in the wellness world are turning to CBD because of its positive effects, including those that help with anxiety and inflammation in the body.

CBD is a powerful tool – used for thousands of years. While the western world has turned it into a villain, CBD has been used to heal many ailments in ways that modern medicine just can't. In the past few years, CBD has been brought back into the mainstream news, mainly because of its effectiveness and the therapeutic properties it contains.

This happened when Charlotte, a little girl who suffered from hundreds of seizures each week, started to take CBD and was almost instantaneously relieved. Since that time, more and more people have started to see the benefits of CBD and have started to use it on their own. In fact, many parents who have exhausted other options for helping their children with various medical concerns have started to go to parts of the world, including Colorado most recently, in order to see whether CBD would be able to help their children.

For some time, only those who were really sick would try to get CBD, and usually only when they had tried all other options. Now, increasing numbers of people are considering CBD for a variety of ailments – some serious – some not.

Despite the growing popularity in cannabis, especially in the form of CBD, many people still have a lot of questions about what this plant is all about and how it can help them feel better. Let's look at what CBD is all about and what it is able to do for your body.

What are some of the ways CBD oil helps my body and mind?

This chemical is known as a modulator, regulator, and an adaptogen. It acts in a fashion that is both dynamic and comprehensive based on the situation you are using it for and the location where it is most needed.

You will quickly find that there are a ton of physiological benefits of using this compound. To start, CBD promotes homeostasis, or balance, in the body. If your body is suffering from some sort of illness or disease because it is imbalanced, which can happen when you are dealing with cancer, inflammation, and a whole host of other diseases.

Homeostasis sets the body in "neutral". CBD oil can kill cancer cells, decrease your blood pressure, and even reduce inflammation that can cause joint and muscle pain.

Some people wonder how CBD oil is able to do what it does. The list that we gave above only talks about a few ways CBD oil can help – and they are all quite different. How is it possible that such a simple compound is able to help out so many different ailments in the body?

The way that CBD oil works has led it to be known as the "Boy Scout Molecule." The reason for the name is because the CBD molecule always knows how to do the right thing based on the situation it confronts. Research has revealed that there are a good 50 mechanisms of action that CBD is able to control, and it is possible for CBD to be a multi-target therapy. This is great news compared to the common analgesic pain medication that only works on one area at a time. CBD gets into the body and works on a variety of things in many different situations.

No matter what is ailing your body, CBD can swoop in and make a difference. This is why it can help one person who is suffering from cancer while also helping someone suffering from anxiety, someone who has issues with inflammation, and even someone with a seizure disorder. And if you are dealing with more than one issue at a time, such as high blood pressure *and* anxiety, it is likely that the CBD molecule will be able to effectively help you with both simultaneously.

Insomnia and anxiety

One of the biggest uses of CBD is to help with anxiety and insomnia. These are both disorders of the brain that cause it to react in ways that may not be seen as normal or regular. Those who deal with anxiety often try to avoid situations that may cause them to overreact. Insomnia is a condition in which the body cannot turn off and let you fall asleep.

Research has shown a significant relationship between CBD, the central nervous system, the endocannabinoid system, and various neurotransmitters in the brain. Even though the CBD part of the plant is not intoxicating, it is able to positively affect your mood. It can also act on the serotonin receptors in the brain, can regulate the GABA regulators that are involved in anxiety, and much more.

There are other products on the market to help with insomnia, but often these have a lot of bad side effects and require the introduction of unnatural chemicals to your body. With the help of CBD, you can enjoy all of the benefits of dealing with your anxiety or insomnia without having to worry about all the usual side effects that come with other products.

What is the Endocannabinoid System and how does it work?

The endocannabinoid system was only discovered a few decades ago. It is complicated because it runs along many different parts of our body. The best way to think of this system is a series of cell receptors matched up with specific molecules that are called "agonists".

To think of it another way, the receptor molecules are like ports. Every time a ship docks, the chemical molecules bind to that "ship" (cell) and all the information and instructions from that vessel are unloaded. It is also similar to a key that fits perfectly and opens a lock.

This system – an inter-connected series of mechanisms is made of three main components including:

- Cells that allow the receipt and the transmission of cannabinoid receptors;
- Specific enzymes tasked with creating or eliminating cannabinoids; and,
- Endocannabinoids, which the body is able to produce naturally and will resemble cannabinoid compounds.

These three parts foster communication inside the body and allow the various biological responses and functions to work well.

The endocannabinoid system is important to homeostasis in the body. In an ideal world, our bodies act in balance and in the proper way through a process known as "homeostasis". However, this homeostasis is constantly being ruined by bad diet, toxins, stressors, and other factors. When this happens, the body does not naturally produce the right number of endocannabinoids and the ones that are produced are not regulated well. The result is disease, illness, and general poor health.

Whenever the balance of the body is compromised, the endocannabinoid system will kick in and try to produce more cannabinoids naturally. They transmit through the body to connect with the cannabinoid receptors that reside on the cells. When the endocannabinoids dock with their cell receptors, they share messages about this change in condition so that the cells can work to adapt and reach homeostasis again.

The endocannabinoid system works with:

- Moderating and boosting brain signals
- Enriching connective tissue
- Regulation of organs and glands
- Influence on the immune system
- Mood
- Pain responses
- Energy levels
- Pleasure and the reward centers inside the brain
- Motor control
- Sleep
- Immune function
- Digestion, appetite, and hunger
- Memory
- Regulating body temperature
- Reproduction and fertility

As previously stated, there are two main variations of the cannabinoid receptors in this system, the CB1 and CB2 receptors. They are separated out because they react uniquely to cannabinoids. The CB1 receptors are found mostly in the central nervous system, which means they will be responsible to certain bodily functions.

The CB2 receptors are found in the peripheral nervous system, the gastrointestinal tract, spleen, and immune system. They not only help with homeostasis, but also help to repair tissue damage and fight inflammation. There are some cells that will contain receptors for CB1 and CB2, with each of them serving a different role in cell function.

The next question is, "What happens when there is a deficiency in the endocannabinoid system?" Scientists have given the label of Clinical Endocannabinoid Deficiency Syndrome, or CEDS, to the state when this system is weakened or compromised because the balance is disrupted. Since these molecules are messengers in the body, any deviation from the norm can result in a host of maladies.

When CEDS occurs, the body cannot produce enough cannabinoids. The individual will lack sufficient messengers to help regulate their systems, making it hard to feel good, to have a good immunity, and more.

Scientists believe that CEDS prohibits the body from producing the correct levels of cannabinoids, meaning the body cannot control various symptoms and making a person more susceptible to disease and illness. Taking more cannabinoids in on a daily basis could help to regulate the body better naturally, at least until the body is able to do it independently.

Cannabinoid supplements have been used for a long time to treat a wide variety of illnesses including:

- Pain
- Seizures
- Epilepsy
- Chronic inflammation
- Depression
- Obesity
- Nausea
- Neurodegenerative diseases
- Insomnia
- Diabetes and high blood sugar
- Glaucoma
- And more

The endocannabinoid system influences almost every part of the body as previously mentioned. It works to keep the body in a constant state of homeostasis, but sometimes things do not work out the way they should. With our modern lifestyles, it is easy to knock the body out of homeostasis; taking cannabinoids can help the body return to balance in ways modern medicines cannot.

Understanding how CBD works with the brain and body

Many people are confused about how the CBD oil works with the body and whether it is going to cause any harm either to the body or the brain.

The ECS is vital to your overall health. It is active to some extent or another in almost all disease states. Since CBD and cannabis target this particular system through different actions, cannabis has applications to a wide variety of diseases.

With research moving forward and looking at the implications of what cannabis is able to do, it is believed that it won't be long before more people understand how cannabis works with the body to help it be more efficient. This is an exciting time; we are just beginning to understand how cannabis works. Many people are excited to learn that they may not have to suffer with many common diseases and illnesses any longer.

Short-term effects of CBD oil

The short-term effects of CBD oil vary based on who takes it and the condition(s) they have. Some people will report relief from very visible maladies (like seizures). Others simply report a better feeling of general wellness, such as feeling less stress or being able to sleep better. Still others tell of reduced inflammation as CBD works with the body's receptors to relieve pain and to reduce swelling.

The way that you feel will depend on the condition you are treating.

If you are dealing with a more serious condition, you will also notice improvements. Sometimes it takes a bit longer to see improvement (based on the type and severity of the condition you face). The good news is that those who take this oil to help with a related health condition report that they feel better even after a short time.

Each person will react differently – just as with any other medicine or regimen. Start with a low dosage and see how you feel. As you progress, you can adjust the amount you ingest. Be as objective as possible – it might be advisable to write down your observations (for accuracy).

The long-term effects of CBD oil

The long-term effects (like short-term) will depend on the disorder you are treating, and your individual make up. To date, research has not uncovered any negative, long-term effects for people using the oil to improve their overall health and wellbeing.

If you are suffering from a disorder such as inflammation, headaches, or seizures, you can take this oil as you determine on a regular, daily basis. Whether you decide to use the oil on a regular or occasional basis, CBD is safe and effective to take for the long-term if needed.

Chapter 4: The Health Benefits of CBD Oil

Many people consider the benefits of CBD oil because they are dealing with health issues and have tried everything else without success. They may have tried all kinds of other treatments and medications, but their symptoms do not diminish – sometimes they get worse. People do not take CBD for fun or for the effects of getting high; they use the oil to improve their health.

Cannabis is an effective treatment for a variety of conditions and diseases and it very often exceeds the performance of traditional medicine. If you are searching for an answer to a whole host of issues and concerned about the side effects of pharmaceuticals, CBD might be the right option for you.

Let's take a look at some of the great health benefits that come with CBD and why it may be a good choice.

Cancer and chemotherapy

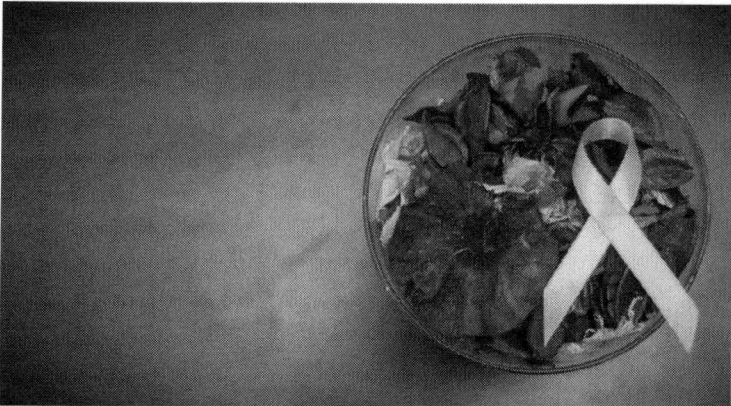

CBD helps patients deal with the effects of chemotherapy. Those who struggle with, or become sick from, chemotherapy can take cannabis and see a decrease in their nausea. This makes it easier to get through the treatments just because you have more energy and can even eat more.

CBD can also elevate your mood. Patients who are feeling down and sad about their diagnoses may find that CBD lifts their spirits. Having a positive attitude is so important for a good treatment outcome.

A group of specialists at the National Cancer Institute reviewed experiments with rhesus monkeys and rodents. The results of these studies implied that CBD has the ability to inhibit the division of cancerous cells, especially when it came to cancers like lymphoma and leukemia. The CBD chemical was also able to lower the probability that the affected tissue would spread over to other parts of the body. In addition, it can increase the effectiveness of the macrophage cells that attack the cancerous cells in the body.

CBD medications could be used as a replacement treatment to chemotherapy altogether. Some patients have been able to take the CBD medications to stop the cancer by inhibiting the cells from dividing and growing. Since the cells can no longer divide, they begin to die. CBD also helps prevent the cancerous cells from moving to other parts of the body. When combined with other treatments, it works to keep the cancer localized and can make healing and recovering much easier.

Heart disease and diabetes

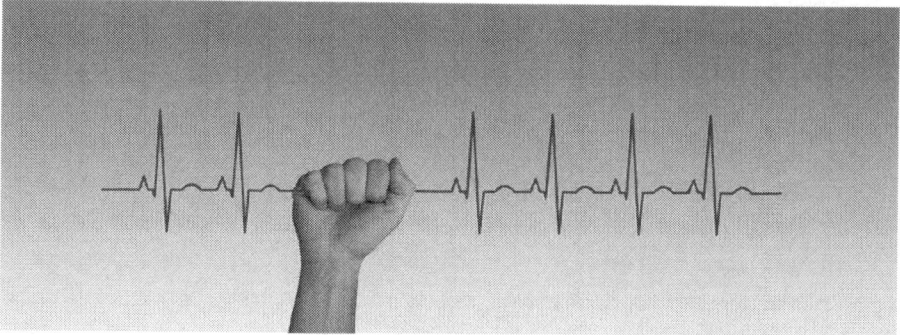

CBD oil carries many anti-inflammatory properties, which we will discuss in more detail later. Consequently, it can help with both diabetes and heart disease. First, because of the anti-inflammatory properties, insulin resistance is reduced, which leads to a better prognosis in many patients by lowering the incidence of dead tissue in the body.

Since CBD was discovered in the 1990s, there has been speculation on its effect on other types of receptors in the body, not just on cannabinoid receptors, and whether it could be manipulated and included in various treatment options for cardiovascular diseases like atherosclerosis.

Speculation led to clinical studies. Researchers at the University of Tel Aviv completed studies that showed a 30 percent increase in blood flow in rodents with areas of dead tissue in the heart muscle.

This is good news for those suffering from either heart disease or diabetes. You will be able to reduce your insulin resistance if you take CBD, which makes it easier to prevent or manage your diabetes, especially if you do it along with a healthy lifestyle and a healthy diet. Additionally, you can keep your heart healthy and reduce the issues that come with areas of dead tissue leading to the heart. You can understand why an increasing number of people are looking to try CBD oil.

Muscle spasms and seizures

One of the main reasons people can acquire CBD (or medical marijuana) legally is for the treatment of muscle spasm disorders. There are many documented cases of children and adults who suffered from extreme seizure disorders, terrible situations where no other treatments had helped, who began to take CBD oil with wonderful results. Their seizures stopped or became very minimal. CBD provided a natural cure.

The information above relates chiefly to epilepsy. The FDA currently allows epilepsy centers throughout the United States to prescribe products that contain CBD to patients, as long as these patients are not responding to classical medication.

A 2015 comprehensive study focusing on Lennox-Gastaut Syndrome and Dravet Syndrome (two very difficult forms of epilepsy) is responsible for the change in treatment protocols. Uncovering the correct treatment and dosage in these two conditions had been very difficult. Children using CBD and marijuana exhibited marked improvement – in some cases, seizures disappeared.

Those who took cannabidiol medication for six months found a decrease between 54 and 67 percent. It is important to note that the CBD oil is effective, but it does not work in every patient. There were some participants in the study above who stopped the treatment after three months because it did not improve their conditions at all.

More studies are needed to demonstrate how and why CBD oil works and to determine why is helps some patients but not others. Still, the future looks promising.

Chronic pain

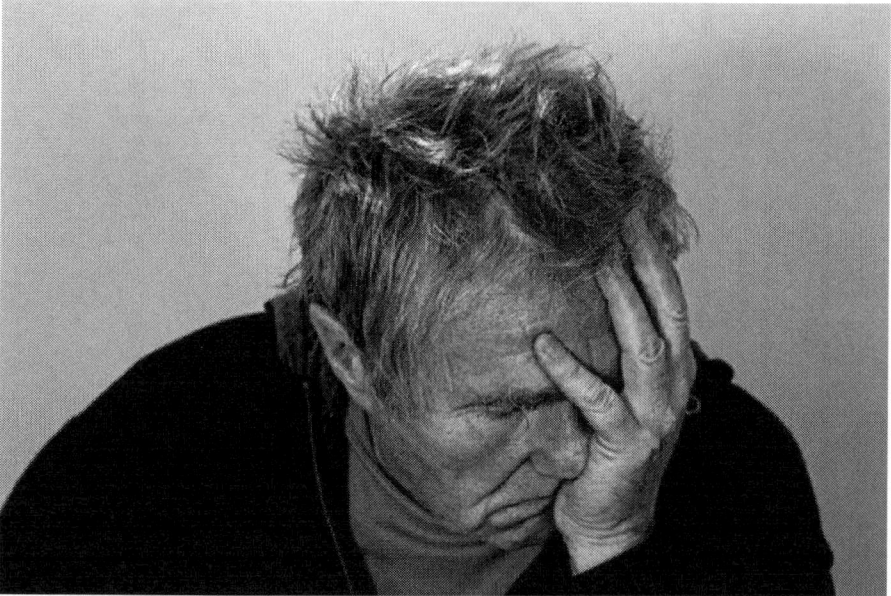

For those suffering from chronic pain, each day can be hard. Chronic pain can make it tough to do even some of the most basic tasks – life sometimes becomes unbearable. Looking for decent chronic pain medications is a challenge. Many drugs also have bad side effects, especially if you take them over the long term. You could even become addicted to these medications.

However, CBD can be a great natural alternative. It works at relieving the chronic pain and many people with such pain found that taking it was a very effective alternative treatment, with limited side effects, that helped them to get their lives back on track.

While cannabis in all forms, including CBD oil, is illegal in most countries, there is a relatively widespread legal provision that allows certain patients to use medical marijuana to help with pain relief. There are certain requirements you must meet to get the medical marijuana legally, but this is a good step in the right direction.

Even though the use of medical marijuana for the treatment of chronic pain is pretty limited at this time, as the population begins to age throughout the world, the incidence of chronic pain will increase. Many elderly people suffer from chronic pain. This growing issue is a matter of public compassion and health.

In 2008, a study looked into the efficacy of cannabinoids other than THC in pain management. It showed that participants tolerated painkillers containing cannabinoids very well, with minimal side effects and without the issue of long-erm toxicity. In addition, when CBD, was combined with opioids, the effect was even more pronounced, and many researchers believe that this is the breakthrough for future in palliative care.

Managing anxiety

Anxiety can take over the life of the sufferer. It is not uncommon for many different people to suffer from anxiety. While everyone feels anxious at some time or another, true anxiety can prove debilitating and drive suffers to extremes as they attempt to avoid any anxiety-producing situation.

Unfortunately, most of the treatment options are not the best. The medications are hard on the body and can have a ton of bad side effects that are sometimes worse than the actual disorder. Some people turn to therapists with varying degrees of success. An improperly trained therapist can make the situation worse.

CBD oil has exhibited some success here. The anxiolytic effect of THC is documented in many different studies and when it is combined with other cannabinoids, such as CBD, it can provide relief. The exact way CBD works to treat anxiety has not yet been ascertained. However, a preliminary study published in 2013 in the *International Neuropsychopharmacology Journal* has set the foundation for more research in the future to show that CBD could be a great treatment for anxiety and for depression in many patients.

This is especially true for those who are dealing with situations that have not improved using more traditional methods. CBD oil is very effective in calming the individual down – to decrease excitement and worry. Since CBD carries no long-term side effects, more and more people are considering it as an option.

Various autoimmune disorders

It is also possible to use CBD and cannabis to deal with a variety of autoimmune disorders. This can be great for people who are dealing with these disorders and who are not able to get regular medication to work for them. Autoimmune disorders can really mess with your life and even if others cannot see what is going on with you, these can be really dangerous and hard to deal with. Those with autoimmune disorders may need to change their diets, their lifestyles, and even go on medication that is harmful and doesn't seem to do much to make them feel better.

CBD oil has a singular mechanism of reducing inflammation in most patients. If you have issues like joint pain or arthritis, this could be your solution. Unlike some of the other medications you may use to treat inflammation, CBD oil does not have the accompanying side effects. You can enjoy the healing benefits in a safe and natural way.

This could change the we deal with autoimmune diseases. Instead of simply managing the pain all of the time, sufferers can take some of this oil and see a vast, almost immediate, improvement. And since there are no side effects, it is a treatment that the patient can use for as long as they need it.

Acne

While this one may not seem as important as some of the others on the list, it is still another health benefit to consider. Acne is a common skin problem that touches almost everyone at one point or another. More than nine percent of the population suffer from it on a regular basis and find that other treatments just do not work.

There are a lot of reasons for acne, including genetics, inflammation under the skin, bacteria, and an overproduction of sebum in the body. Based on some recent studies, it is possible that CBD oil could treat acne mostly due to the oil's ability to reduce inflammation. CBD is effective at reducing the amount of sebum production in the body, which can mean less acne as well.

One study found that CBD could prevent the sebaceous gland cells from secreting excessive sebum while also preventing the activation of "pro-acne" agents like inflammation cytokines. Another study had some similar findings and concluded that CBD may be a safe and efficient way to treat acne, especially if you have tried other methods without success.

Antibacterial

There have been several studies demonstrating how CBD oil exhibits antibacterial properties. One such study, performed at the Italian Piemonte University and later published in 2008, implied that all types of cannabinoids the immune system fight bacteria.

Even though all of cannabinoids are good at helping with this, it seems there are five cannabinoids, including CBD, that the study focused on because of their antibiotic resistant properties. Considering that a lot of people are overusing antibiotics and are now resistant to them, it is nice to think there may be a healthy and effective alternative.

Reduces inflammation in the body

One of the biggest reasons some people choose to go with this treatment is because the chemicals contained in CBD reduce inflammation in the body. CBD enhances bone growth, making them stronger and more resistant to inflammation, osteoporosis and other disorders.

There are even some studies, most notably the ones from the University of Tel Aviv, that discovered rats given CBD supplements recovered from fractures up to 40 percent faster compared to those who did not take the supplement. CBD oil may provide relief for these conditions and accelerate the healing process.

Headaches

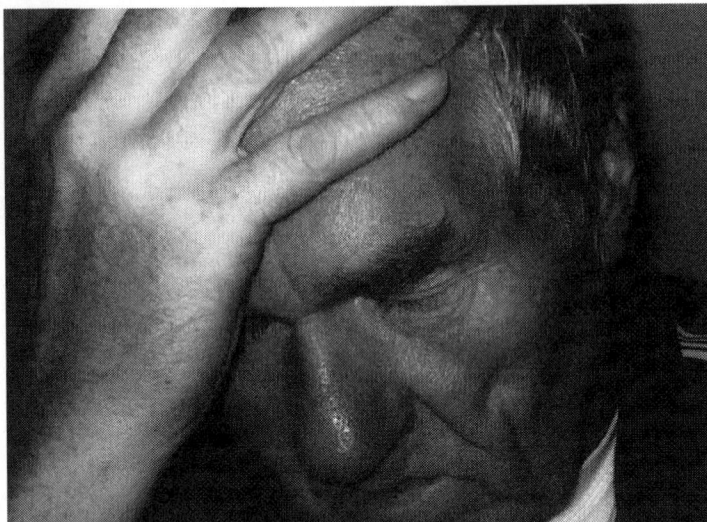

Headache sufferers may benefit from the use of CBD and cannabis. Most of those who use CBD oil for headaches have been dealing with debilitating pain for a long time. They may have tried a lot of different medications throughout the years and are still not seeing any benefits. These headaches negatively impact quality of life and can limit the activities in which they participate.

CBD oil works with the transmitters in the brain to alleviate pain. CBD can be very effective even if other treatments or medications have not worked in the past. If you are tired of dealing with headaches and nothing else seems to work for you, then it may be time to try some CBD to see if that can give you a little bit of relief.

Eating disorders

In some cases, cachexia and anorexia patients can use CBD and cannabis as an effective and safe treatment. Cachexia is a severe disorder that involves a dangerous amount of weight loss. This is a bit different than some of the other eating disorders that you may encounter because rather than the patient purposely trying to lose the weight, this dangerous weight loss is brought on by some sort of disease, such as Alzheimer's (where the patient may forget to eat), cancer, or AIDS.

In 2011, a study in Germany involving over 100 people proved that patients who were on a placebo were able to lose about 80 percent more weight each week compared to those who received a cannabinoid cocktail. This shows that the CBD oil may be able to prevent weight loss or help you to keep on or gain weight if needed.

Additionally, CBD oil can be used as a form of treatment for those who are suffering from a variety of eating disorders, including anorexia nervosa. While gaining weight, the CBD user also benefits from the calming and mental-improvement qualities of the oil.

Tourette's Syndrome

Tourette's Syndrome affects about one percent of the population. The cause of this disorder is unknown, but while more and more people are diagnosed with this disorder each year, most treatment options are lacking. According to Kristen R. Muller-Vahl, M.D., current treatments are unsatisfactory, which leads to more interest in using cannabis and other holistic treatments.

Muller-Vahl describes two clinical studies conducted in 2002. One of these studies involved giving 12 patients one dose of THC. Two weeks later, they were given a placebo. Seventy-five percent of the participants reported positive effects from the first round.

The second study had 24 participants, all of whom were affected by tics from TS. With this study it was reported that THC was able to reduce tics in patients. in addition, neither study showed that there were serious adverse effects to taking cannabis for this disorder. Muller-Vahl suggests that when the major Tourette's Syndrome drugs do not work for patients, then using medical marijuana can be an effective treatment.

PTSD

You can also use *Cannabis r* to help deal with symptoms of PTSD. Most sufferers of this use the cannabis as a way to self-medicate, so studies on it are not as prevalent as for other disorders. Many of those who have PTSD find it difficult to cope with the unpleasant and intense symptoms. Issues like nightmares, anger, hyperarousal, sleep problems, and intrusive memories and thoughts are common and can interfere with the daily functioning of these individuals.

Taking one of the strains of cannabis can help provide quick relief from these symptoms. It can get rid of the anxiety and help the sufferer relax. It may not address the root of the problem and those suffering from PTSD will need to take other treatment actions, however cannabis can help to relax the patient. Once in this more beneficial relaxed state, patients are in a better position to be treated with other therapies and methods either alongside of or without cannabis.

Period pain

It is believed that cannabis can even help with monthly period pain. A 2002 review described tonics (made as early as 2000 BC) that were made from beer, mint, saffron, and hemp seed and then given to women to help ease their pain during difficult childbirth. In 1596, a medical text from China listed that cannabis flowers were a good way to ease symptoms that women experienced during menstruation. It is even said that Queen Victoria used the herb to receive relief from painful cramping and it was common for Victorian doctors to prescribe this as well.

Today, even with the issues of legality of the herb in most of the world, women are still turning to cannabis in order to self-treat problems they have with the womb. This includes those who use it to help with period cramps, pregnancy complications, bloating, and more.

Boosting athletic performance

While some people still envision cannabis users as stoners who are lazy and won't get off the couch, there is evidence that it can be used to improve athletic performance. In fact, it can be viewed as a tool for use in sports medicine. There are not many available studies on the subject at this moment (since cannabis is largely an illegal substance), but there is a lot of anecdotal evidence stating how cannabis increases concentration, confidence, and stamina during athletic activities.

Cannabis can be used to boost any kind of athletic performance and long-distance runners are a good example of how this can work. Many long-distance runners have shared how cannabis has helped them to have more endurance and positive mental focus while training. Snowboarders and skiers talk about how this drug can help them to concentrate and lose their fear and anxiety when they are on the slopes.

In addition, weight lifters mention how cannabis lessens the amount of pain that they feel when working on a heavy lift. Cannabis talk may even make it onto the football field. Many believe that it could help players cope with off-field pain better than taking traditional painkillers and that it could help treat traumatic brain injury.

Some of the strains that could help with athletic performance include:

- Casey Jones
- Bruce Banner BX 2.0
- Lemon haze
- Sour diesel
- Bubba kush
- Durban poison
- OG Kush

Hepatitis C

There is some research suggesting that cannabis could offer therapeutic benefits to those who are suffering from HCV and other diseases of the liver. Major cannabinoids that are found in cannabis bind and influence the CB1 and CB2 receptors in the endocannabinoid system. The CB2 is responsible for reducing inflammation in the body and can be beneficial on alcoholic fatty liver, liver injury, regeneration, fibrosis, and hepatic inflammation.

Patients have found some success with taking cannabis to help treat the symptoms they experience with Hepatitis C and the nausea that can come from some of the treatments of this disease.

Fibromyalgia

Fibromyalgia sufferers may be able to get more relief from medical marijuana than they can from any of the three prescription drugs approved by the FDA. According to the National Institutes of Health, there are roughly five million Americans who suffer from fibromyalgia, a condition that can include symptoms such as lack of sleep, depression, headaches, fatigue, and deep tissue pain. Many respondents to a survey from the National Institutes of Health say that they have tried at least one prescription medication for their symptoms, and quite a few had tried all three.

Sixty to 70 percent of patients agreed that these prescriptions did not work and that the limited relief did not warrant the side effects.

However, 62 percent of those who tried cannabis to treat their symptoms said that it was very effective, and another 33 percent said that it helped a little. Compared to prescription medications where most people saw no relief, only five percent of those who tried cannabis said that it did not work.

Schizophrenia

There is currently an experimental cannabis drug used to treat schizophrenia. This drug was developed by GQ Pharmaceuticals Plc, a UK-based business, and was found to be superior to a placebo in mid-stage trials. The drug, cannabidiol, was tested on 88 patients, all of whom experienced schizophrenia but had not responded to anti-psychotic medication in the past.

During the trial, the patients continued to take their medications while some received a placebo and other received the cannabidiol. This study found that those who took the cannabis experienced fewer episodes of schizophrenia compared to those that took the placebo. GW has plans to test this drug on other health-related issues including pain from cancer and epilepsy.

CBD in mother's breast milk

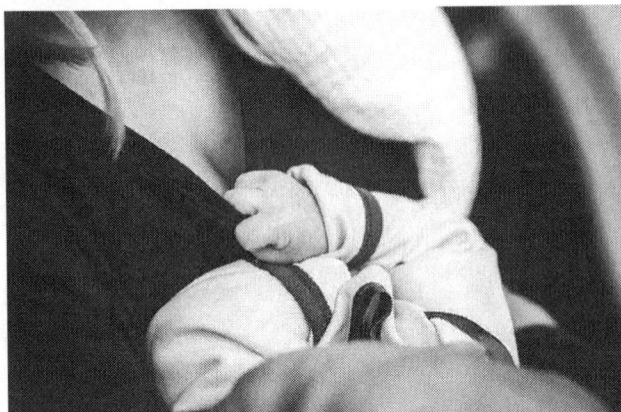

Emerging research shows that cannabinoids found in the breast milk are important to the development and growth of the human infant. These chemicals can help to jumpstart the appetite of the baby because the mother produces cannabinoids naturally, which ultimately promote the healthy development in the baby.

Studies have shown that two endocannabinoids, anandamide and 2-arachidonyl glycerol, are both found in the human embryo. In the beginning, the anandamide works to help regulate the appetite and one's pleasure and reward systems. It begins in low concentrations in the embryo and then will slowly increases until the baby is mature. The 2-arachidonyl glycerol works the opposite way.

The baby, when born, will not produce CBD on their own. Babies rely on the mother's milk to provide them with this chemical to keep their appetite up and to aid in their development. If the baby has trouble gaining weight and doesn't have much of an appetite, the mother may want to talk to her doctor about including some CBD oil in her diet. This chemical would then be passed on to the baby through the milk and could help the baby to increase appetite and in turn, gain more weight.

CBD for beauty and anti-aging

Many have decided to start using CBD to help fight the effects of aging and to make them look younger and more vibrant. CBD oil is full of great anti-oxidants and vitamins that can protect your body from the harmful effects of free radicals. It can even protect you from the sun. If your body is exposed to too many of the above, over time your skin will start to show it.

Using a topical form of CBD can help to keep the skin looking good. The high concentration of vitamin A in the oil, which is crucial to the growth and differentiation of skin cells, helps your skin look amazing. In addition, the vitamin D inside the oil combines with vitamin A in order to prevent the skin from getting flaky and dry. It is an extremely good natural moisturizer.

Other benefits

Because of the rising popularity of CBD, many new studies are being conducted to explore how multi functional CBD oil can be and how much it can do to keep the human body healthy. While many people may still be worried about trying out this treatment because of its association with cannabis, it won't be long before it becomes more of a staple in our culture. Some of the other benefits you could receive with the use of this treatment includes:

- Antipsychotic effects: Some studies are suggesting that using CBD could help people who are suffering from schizophrenia and some other mental disorders. It is able to do this by reducing the psychotic symptoms of the sufferer.

- A treatment for substance abuse: CBD has been shown to modify the circuits in the brain that are closely related to drug addiction. In rats, CBD reduced dependence on morphine while also reducing heroin seeking behavior.
- Anti-tumor effects: In animal and test tube studies, CBD has demonstrated the ability to stop tumors. It can even help to prevent the spread of various cancers like lung, colon, brain, prostate, and breast.

As you can see, there are a ton of health benefits with CBD oil. Whether you need help with an autoimmune disorder, want to improve your heart, have issues with headaches, and more, you will find that adding CBD to your lifestyle will make a profound difference in how you think and feel.

Chapter 5: Are There Any Negatives to Using CBD Oil?

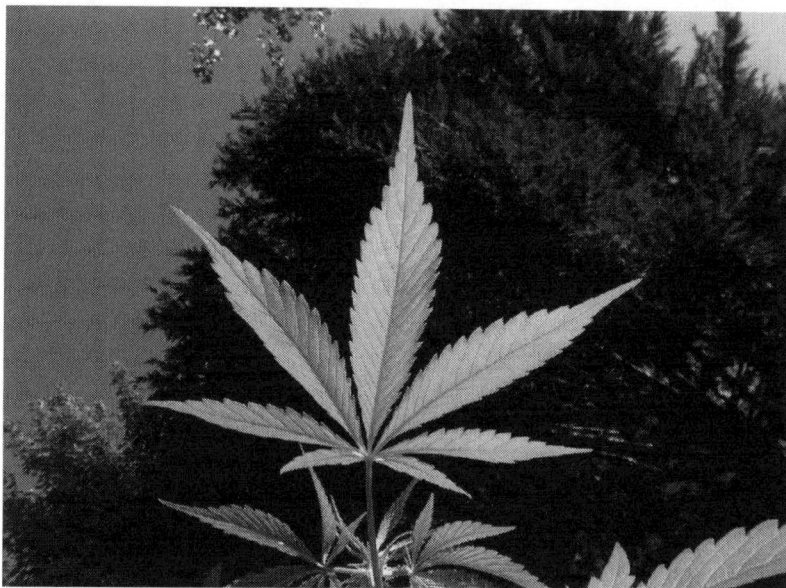

The last chapter spent a lot of time talking about all the great uses that you can get out of CBD as a treatment. You are able to work on your heart health, reduce the issues that come with diabetes, help with cancer as a treatment and as a way to keep nausea away, and so much more. With all the good benefits, especially for many patients who have tried other things and not seen success, it seems like CBD is the miracle that they have been seeking.

CBD and cannabis have always offered a wide range of useful applications. With changing attitudes, more and more people are recognizing the benefits of CBD and medical marijuana.

Still, many people ask whether there are some bad side effects that come with CBD and taking its oil. We talked about this a bit throughout the other chapters, but now it is time to take a closer look at CBD oil and determine whether it is safe for people to use and what, if any, side effects it carries.

The biggest drawback comes from the negative connotations associated with cannabis. Because the authorities and the government in the United States have decided that CBD, as well as all other parts of the cannabis plant, are bad, it has been regarded this way by the general public for a long time. Even though CBD oil, as well as other parts of the cannabis plant, are safe and effective, many people still see them as potentially harmful.

Since the government sees all cannabis as an illegal drug, there are no clear regulations regarding CBD and its products. There are no regulations concerning how it should be produced and handled. This can cause some tension and uncertainty about the options of CBD oil on the market. If you are trying to use CBD oil for personal health reasons, you may be confused.

When purchasing CBD in any form, do your research and ensure that you go to a reputable seller. You want a high-quality product and one that is not full of other things that could cause problems. You also have to be careful about where you get CBD oil because, with all the different names and minimal regulation in place, it is possible that you could get a product that does contain psychoactive THC and you might not get the benefits you desire.

Some studies show that CBD oil brings on a cotton mouth sensation in some patients. Many believe the issue comes from the proximity of the cannabinoid receptors to the submandibular glands, which are responsible for producing saliva. For some people, this means that the production of saliva can be affected. Not everyone experiences this problem. There is no risk to your health – you will just feel thirsty and may need to drink some more water.

Pay attention to the dosage that you are taking. CBD oil can worsen uncontrollable muscle movements and tremors if taken in high doses. If taken at the right dosage, however, it can help with these types of issues, including Parkinson's.

Always start with a very low dosage and build up until you reach the amount that provides you with relief. This ensures you get all of the good benefits that come with the CBD oil, without having to worry about taking too much or potentially experiencing any adverse effects.

Another reason to watch the dosage is because CBD can sometimes stop the activity of a few enzymes found inside the liver. These enzymes, known as the P450 enzymes, are responsible for metabolizing the drugs or medications that you commonly use. If you are not on any medications, then this is probably not a big issue. If you are on medication though, you may want to talk to your doctor before taking CBD oil to see how that could affect the way that the other medication works.

Some of the other side effects that you will need to watch out for include:

- Lightheadedness: This one ties into the next and often people will feel it because their blood pressure decreases. Be careful about the amount that you take each day and try having a cup of tea or some coffee to help get the blood pressure back up.

- Low blood pressure: Taking too much CBD oil for your condition can result in a lower blood pressure. This will usually happen soon after taking the CBD. This is a temporary side effect, however if you are already taking drugs for your blood pressure, you want to be careful. Always talk with your doctor before you get started using CBD.

- Fatigue: This treatment can cause drowsiness, but again, this usually happens when the dosage of CBD is too high. If you feel drowsy when taking it, you need to be careful when driving or using machinery and you may need to consider reducing your dosage. In most cases, as long as the dosage is appropriate, it will help you feel full of energy and more awake.

Remember that these side effects are not going to be the same for everyone. Some people will experience mild cases of these side effects, but most people take CBD oil and (as long as they stay within the dosage that is correct for them) will be perfectly fine. Listen to your body and be careful, albeit this is the same advice you would follow no matter what kind of supplement you use.

Chapter 6: How to Make CBD Oil

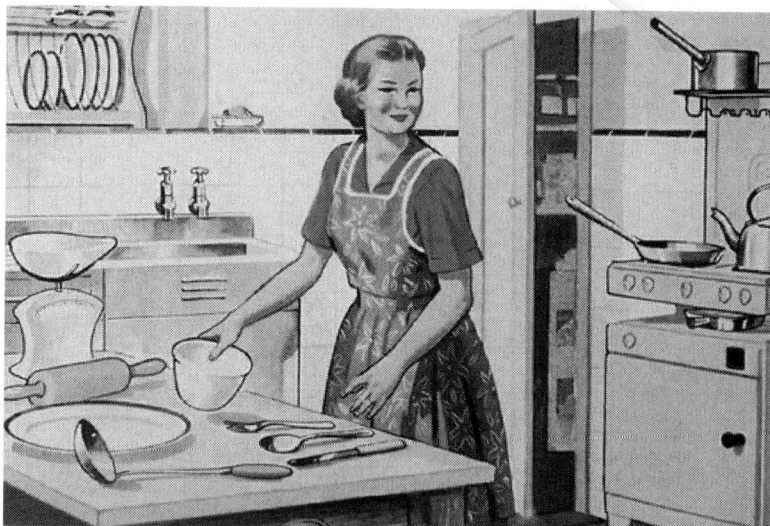

CBD oil is quickly growing in popularity. Many people are starting to see that there is a difference between the various parts of the cannabis plant and are hearing more and more about all the medical benefits coming out about CBD and the products that are made using it. Because of this, many people are interested in learning more about CBD oil and how they can acquire it.

Learning how to make your own CBD is one of the best ways to understand how it works, impacts the body and even how it differs from the THC found in marijuana.

The three methods of making CBD oil

There are a few different methods of making CBD oil. The method you choose is going to vary based on the type of CBD oil you want to make and the method that seems the best for you. The three different methods to extract CBD oil from the cannabis plant include:

> The CO2 method. By pushing CO2 through the plant, using low temperatures and high pressures, you will get the CBD in its purest form. Because of the way this method works, it is often seen as the best, as well as the safest, if you want to extract CBD cleanly. This method will help you to remove harmful substances, such as chlorophyll and it doesn't leave a residue.

  Any oil made by extracting CBD in this manner has a cleaner taste compared to the other two methods. That being said, it is a lot more expensive compared to the other two methods, which is why some people do not choose to go with the CO2 method.

> The Ethanol method. CBD is sometimes extracted with the help of high-grain alcohol. The biggest issue with this one is that while it proves a bit more cost effective than the other options, if made incorrectly then this method could potentially harm some of the beneficial natural oils that come with CBD, which may make it a bit less effective for treatment in some of the illnesses and diseases. If made with care however then this method will work well.

> The Oil method. This one is growing in popularity, so it is likely that when you purchase CBD, it will have been produced this way. This method involves extraction using a type of carrier oil. There are a few options you can choose from, but olive oil is the most commonly used. The reason this method is so popular is because you get some of the nutritional value from the carrier oil and it is also safe and free of those unwanted residues that can ruin the oil.

Let's look at an easy and cost-effective method in more detail.

The Ethanol Method.

Ingredients:

- 30g of ground buds (the dried flower heads or buds of the cannabis plant after they have been ground in a grinder or mortar and pestle)
- Grain alcohol or other food-safe, high % alcohol

You will need:

- Medium size glass, ceramic or metal mixing bowl
- Sieve,
- Medium size catchment container
- Double boiler (a set of two pots that are stacked together with space between them)
- Wooden or metal spoon, silicon spatula, funnel, plastic syringe

Time: Around 45 mins

How to make your oil:

Put the ground buds into the mixing bowl and slowly add the alcohol until it covers the buds. Gently stir for 5 minutes. Filter the solution through the sieve and into the catchment container.

Place the remaining residue in the sieve back into the mixing bowl and again add alcohol and stir as before. Then once again, sieve the mixture into the catchment bowl along with your first batch.

Pour the contents of the catchment bowl into the double boiler and gently bring to the boil. Reduce the heat and let it slowly simmer away the alcohol and stir gently for around 15 minutes. to prevent it sticking to the pan. Once all the alcohol has evaporated scrape the pan with the spatula.

Now place some of the concentrated oil into small dark airtight bottles or dosage containers before it cools and becomes thicker. You can use the plastic syringe to do this or use the opposite end of a metal spoon or fork. Olive, coconut or vegetable oil can then be added to the bottle to dilute the mixture. This last part can be tricky as you want to do this while the concentrated oil is still warm. The quality and strength of your oil will largely depend on the plant used and how well the oil has been produced. This oil can then be consumed. As always be careful with your dosage, especially when you start using a new product.

Getting the CBD oil from hemp rather than medical marijuana

It is possible to get the CBD oil from either the hemp plant or from medical marijuana. However, there are some differences in the oil you get depending on which plant you use. The main difference between getting the CBD oil from hemp compared to getting it from medical marijuana is the amount of THC and the amount of CBD you will get in the final product. Let's take a closer look at both of these compounds and then look at what you are going to get out of the two different plants.

THC has been associated with making users high, which sometimes turns out fine, but many users find that they have negative experiences or side effects from using the THC. There are quite a few psychological disorders associated with prolonged heavy use of THC; another reason it is illegal in most parts of the country.

Why is this important?

Because of the common misconceptions that come with medical marijuana and hemp, it is important understand the differences between THC and CBD and why one is healthier for you when compared to the other.

CBD, as we have discussed previously, is a cannabinoid that our brains have been wired to accept. There are already some special receptor sites in the brain where the CBD cannabinoid can bind including in the immune system and various organs. When cannabinoids, including CBD, start to bind to these special receptor sites, they exert some influence over the functioning or the activity of whatever that particular receptor is controlling.

Research has shown that CBD can interact with these receptor sites in a beneficial way. Rather than interfering and making it harder to functions efficiently or damaging these receptor sites, CBD benefits the receptor site and whatever it is controlling. In fact, adding in CBD to your daily diet can make a positive impact on your general well-being and your health even if you do not have a major health condition.

Chapter 7: How to use CBD oil?

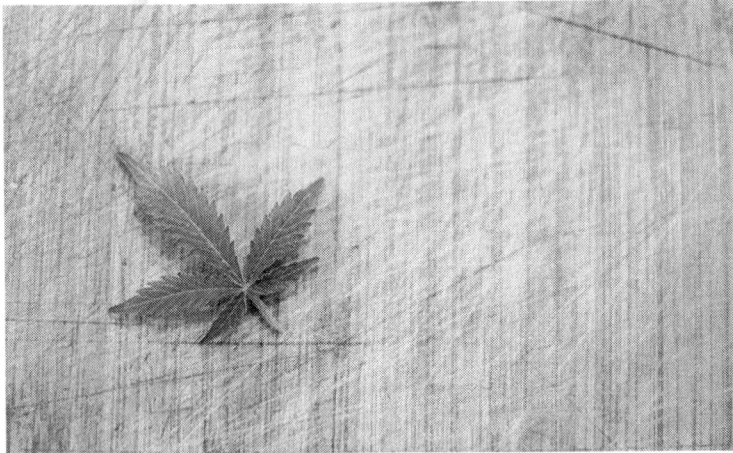

There are a few different methods you can use when it comes to taking your CBD oil. The method we discussed earlier was simply to keep the oil in a jar and consume it when you are ready. There are several options for how you can take this medicine to get the benefits we have discussed. The method you choose will often depend on personal preferences and the disorder you want to treat. Some of the options you have for ingesting CBD include:

Tinctures

The most common way to use CBD is a tincture. Compared to the other products, tinctures are considered the purest application of CBD because the manufacturers do not do any separate processing of the oil. There are a few brands that will add some flavoring to the tinctures. This simply makes it easier for some customers to take the chemical but doesn't change the purity of the product.

A dropper typically holds 1ml of liquid. If you know how many milliliters are in a CBD tincture, you can then use this simple formula to work out how much CBD is in its dropper:

Total CBD in the Bottle ÷ Number of Millileters in the Bottle will give you the MGs of CBD in the Dropper

A typical example would be a 30ml CBD tincture that has 1500MG of CBD: Therefore 1500 ÷ 30 = 50MG of CBD per dropper. Now if you required a dosage of CBD at 25MG, and a single dropper of that 1500MG tincture contains 50MG, you'd simply fill the dropper halfway.

To take you simply put a few drops either on or under the tongue. The dosage will range from 100mg to 1000mg, so start out small and then build up to the amount that you need. The biggest issue with using a tincture is that they get messy if you spill any of the drops. Some people are not comfortable using tinctures.

A tincture is most effective if you do not swallow all the liquid right away. You should work to ingest as much of it as you can sub-bilingually. Place the drops along the cheeks or under the tongue and then leave them there, without swallowing, for as long as you can for the best results.

Concentrates

A CBD concentrate is the strongest dosage of CBD. In fact, it could contain up to 10 times the concentration compared to other similar CBD products. Some people like to take the concentrate because, when compared to a tincture, the concentrate is more convenient. It only takes a few seconds to consume and some will find it a more convenient method.

The biggest negative to working with a concentrate is that it typically is not flavored. The natural flavor is hard to swallow for some users. Some beginners also don't like he concentrates because the syringe shape is intimidating.

For the most part, the CBD concentrates are popular with customers. Concentrates have a high potency and are easy to take so you can get your dosage quicker. To take a CBD concentrate, simply place it under your tongue and along the cheeks and then let it slowly dissolve.

Capsules

Another option you can choose is a capsule. This one is often considered the easiest method to use because you simply take the CBD as a supplement, just like you would take your daily multivitamin. The capsules are easier to take compared to the other two methods, and if you are already taking other supplements, you can easily add the CBD pills to this daily regimen.

The capsules offer between 10 and 25mg of CBD. Since each capsule already offers a set amount, you will find this is one of the easiest ways to keep track of how much you are taking. The pills can sometimes present issues if you want to change your dosage. Some people deal with this by using capsules along with some other types of CBD products, like a tincture, so that they can adjust and control the amount they take.

Capsules are convenient. You just take one, or as many as needed, with water each day to get the desired dosage and results.

Topicals

It is becoming more common to see CBD in topicals, such as lip balms, salve, and lotions. These products deliver great skin benefits. Topicals help with a whole host of things such as a cancer treatment, anti-aging treatment, psoriasis, acne, inflammation, and even chronic pain.

If you want to use topical products, look for the keywords on the product label. Look for *micellization, encapsulation*, or *Nano-technology* of CBD. This shows that the solution can carry the CBD through your dermal layers to provide relief, rather than just keeping it on the skin. Using the CBD infused topical layers are meant to help more with joint or skin-related issues.

To use topicals that are infused with CBD, just follow the same rules as you would with other body care products. Use it as necessary on the area of need. You can apply it generously to any area of the body that would benefit from this topical solution.

Sprays

Most CBD users stay away from the sprays because they have the weakest concentration compared to the other types of CBD products. Most concentrations found in these sprays will range from 1 to 3mg, which is not very high. And when you compare them to the other oral products, it is really hard to measure the exact amount that you take each day because the sprays are inconsistent.

The reason some people will go with the sprays comes from the ease of carrying the product – especially on the road. If you are traveling, it is much easier to spray some of the CBD into your mouth compared to using a concentrate or a tincture. You may need to spray a few times to get any effects though because the concentration is so low in these sprays.

To use, just spray one serving of the bottle straight into your mouth. Each type of spray will be different, so look for the serving size on the label. The serving size will usually be somewhere between two and three sprays. You can use these sprays as needed or simply on a daily basis.

Vapes

Some people choose to ingest their CBD oil through vapes. Based on some reviews from those who have tried it, ingesting the CBD through vapes, vaporizing or smoking CBD vape oil seems to have lower effects compared to some of the other methods that we have discussed. However, others say that vaporizing has fewer drawbacks compared to taking CBD orally.

Smoking CBD can be a good method because you are able to adjust the dosage pretty easily and take it more or less based on how you are feeling. To take CBD by vape, you will just need a vaporizer, a vape pen, or an e-cigarette. Then, you add in some heat, inhale the amount of vape oil that you want through the device, and enjoy.

Edibles

For some people, going with the options above can prove difficult. They may need more relief than they can get with a topical solution. Some may not like the taste of the chemical, even if there are added flavors to the product. They may not be interested in smoking the chemical, so vaping is out of the question. And sometimes you just want to try something different and see how it works.

For these individuals, edibles may be the best option. Edibles are any type of food containing the oil. You can technically add the CBD to any meal or snack that you make. This helps to mask the flavor. Many people like to add the oil to a dessert to make it taste better, but you can also go with other options.

Later, there are several different recipes to try if you want to consume the CBD as an edible. These include options for pantry goods, breakfasts, main meals, and desserts and snacks. You can mix and match the options that you want to use to get your daily dosage.

Remember, edibles take a bit longer to get the relief. The oil has to go through your digestive tract before absorbs into your bloodstream. This can take up to three hours so clearly it is not as fast as some of the other options that are absorbed directly. But for some people, this is the best option to get their dosage of CBD.

Other options

The options above are some of the most popular forms of taking CBD oil and most of them can work well in getting your required daily dose. There are a few other options you can choose from including:

- CBD gums
- CBD patches
- Gel pen

Edibles do seem to be the most popular method of consumption. This is because they offer a tasty and enjoyable way to take CBD compared to the other options, however the main issue with edibles is that unless you are making your own or you make single servings, it is hard to determine consistency.

All of the methods of taking CBD that are listed above can be very effective. Experiment and choose the method that works the best for you. If taste is important to you, then using a tincture or an edible may be the best. If you want to take it along with your other daily vitamins, then a capsule is the best option. All of the methods are going to work to help you feel better; you just have to use your personal preference to determine which one you will use.

Chapter 8: How to Purchase CBD Oil

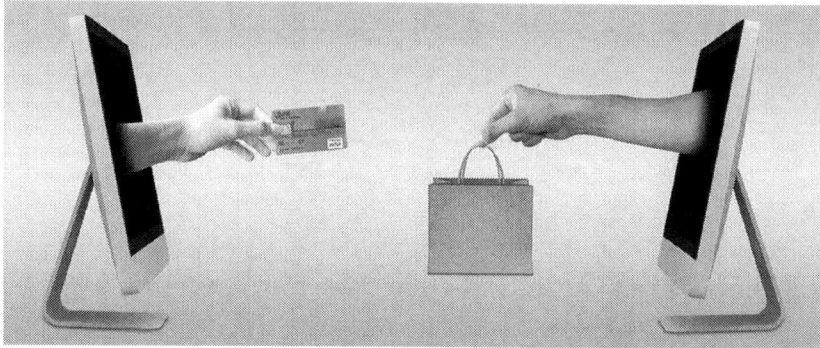

If you are intrigued by the different health benefits that come with CBD oil, and you are interested in giving it a try, the first question you may have is how to purchase the product? The steps are pretty simple, so let's take a look at how to get started!

How to know you are getting a high-quality product?

It is important that you order high-quality CBD oil if you want to gain the maximum health benefits. There are a lot of people trying to get into this market. Many companies will provide high quality oil to the consumer, but others will just look to make a quick buck in a booming trade. Luckily, there are a few things you can look for to ensure that you are getting the best CBD oil possible.

Consider the source

Look first at the oil's source. Hemp that comes from China is a common choice because it usually costs less, allowing suppliers to offer it for less money (and a larger profit). If you want high-quality oil, find a supply from Australia, the United States, or Europe. This sometimes results in a higher price, but it is definitely worth it.

Petroleum-free processing

The oil's extraction method is very important. A chemical-free, cold CO2 extraction method gets the most CBD possible out of the cannabis plant. It is sometimes more expensive, so some producers will not use this method, but it is important to go with this option because it uses safer solvents and ensure that you get a pure and potent extract. It is also non-toxic and eco-friendly.

Check out independent lab results

If you want to make sure that a product is safe and effective to use, check if there are any independent lab results about the product. Not all companies can provide these lab results, but if you can find these, they will give you some reassurance that the CBD is safe to take and higher in quality.

A THC level that is lower than .03%

The highest quality of CBD oil contains HC levels lower than .03%. This ensures that you get all the good effects from the CBD and none of the unwanted one. You may find some options that are a bit higher and they are probably still pretty good for you. But, if you want the highest quality, try to go with options that keep the THC low.

Look for the hemp oil extract using the whole plant

Good quality oils use the whole plant CBD oil. This means that the oil is taken from all of the plant, including the stalks, seeds, and stem. It also includes more than just the CBD inside it such as sugars, secondary cannabinoids, flavonoids, and terpenes. These compounds are believed to work well together to heighten the effect that the CBD has on the body. While some manufacturers only offer CBD from certain parts of the plant, the best quality oil is going to include extracts from the whole plant.

Where to find a good supplier

You could buy from your local dispensary if you have one. Alternatively finding a good online supplier isn't difficult. There are a few things to consider. First, determine the method you want to use when taking the CBD oil. Look at some of the methods we talked about above to help you decide. Some suppliers will offer more than one type of CBD. Knowing the method you want to use can help to trim the number of suppliers you consider.

You also want to take a look at the price of the products. Be careful about the lower priced option. These have usually added things in their mixtures, or they may dilute the oil, so it is barely useful. Compare prices and shop wisely.

Always take a look at the reviews of the company. CBD oil is really popular and while there are many legitimate companies to purchase from, there are also many people jumping into this market just to make money. They do not necessarily provide a good quality product. If you read through the reviews of any company you are considering, it should not take long to figure out which companies are legitimate and which ones are not.

Figuring out the dosage that you should take for your own personal needs

How much will you need to take each day? Each person is going to be different and sometimes, if you take too much, it could get the opposite effects to what you seek.

Just because one person can take a large dose does not mean that you need to take as much, and just because someone gets relief with just a tiny bit doesn't mean you are doing something wrong if you take a larger dose. Starting out small can help you determine exactly how much you need to take. You can always increase your dosage to fit your needs.

To help you determine how much you should start with, here are some guidelines:

- For general health, take 2.5 to 15mg of CBD by mouth each day.
- To treat issues with chronic pain, take 2.5 to 20 mg of CBD by mouth each day.
- To treat sleeping disorders, take 40 to 160 mg of CBD by mouth each day.

As you can see, there is quite a range in the amounts, so how are you supposed to figure out the right dose for you? If you have never tried CBD in the past, there are a few things that you can consider as you make your decision. Each person will find that their dosage is different, so you will want to be careful and ensure you are taking the right amount for your needs.

Some general guidelines to follow include:

- Start out small: When you first get started with CBD, regardless of the condition you are trying to heal, it is always best to start out small. In fact, go with the smallest dose possible. You never know how you are going to react to this supplement and since it is so new, you want to be able to learn how your body responds to the supplement before you increase the dosage. Try it out at that dosage for a few days and if you feel that it is not quite doing the job, then add a little more of the CBD to your regime. As soon as you feel that the dosage is right and is relieving you of the pain or discomfort, then maintain that dose and monitor the situation.

- Pay attention to size and weight of a user. The right dose is going to vary between someone who is small and someone who is bigger. If you are pretty small, such as short or underweight, start out with a very low dose of CBD. If you are a larger person, then you will want to try out a bit more of the oil to see how it goes. With CBD, it is easy to add just a few milligrams to the dosage.

- Talk to a medical professional: If you are dealing with medical conditions, or you are on any type of medication, it is best to talk with your health care professional before you consume the CBD. There are some medications that do not work well with CBD, or which may become less potent when you take CBD and you want to make sure that this does not affect you in a negative manner. A health care professional will be able to answer your questions about CBD and can tell you which doses are the most beneficial based on your personal medical history.

Always remember that CBD is going to react differently in each person, so be careful. Even though it is safe and effective to use, you obviously do not want to suffer any potential adverse effects by using too much. Follow the suggestions that are listed above when you first start adding CBD oil to your daily routine and you will soon find what works best for you.

Is there the "perfect" dosage for everyone?

The amount of CBD you should take for optimum results depends on the type you get, the strain, and how high the concentration of CBD is in the bottle. A typical dosage can be as little as a few milligrams of CBD oil to a gram or more.

Let's look at a typical example. For someone who weighs around 150 pounds, the minimum initial dose is 3mg. The average dose for a person of this size is 10mg, but if you can take less than this, that is best. However, the absolute maximum you should take each day (at 150 pounds) is 63 drops. If you are not experiencing any meaningful results with this amount, it may be time to try out a different method unless this has been specifically prescribed by your doctor.

This is just an example of the recommended dosage. You can find more detailed calculators online that will give you recommendations based on how much you weigh and the particular product and strain of CBD you purchase. Having said that the above guidelines are a fairly accurate starting point. Also, please refer to the charts at the end of this book for dosage relevant to body weight.

How long do the effects last?

When you take CBD in any form, it will stay in your system between three to five days. The length of stay depends on the amount you took – and absorption rates vary among people. If you are going to complete a drug test or anything similar, it is important to note that the CBD, even if you just take it only a few times, may register on the test.

Even though the CBD can stay in your system for a few days, the effects are going to last between three to four hours for most people. If you are using CBD to help with common ailments like the ones we have discussed, you may need to take it a few times a day to keep receiving the benefits.

Does the price make a difference?

When shopping for CBD oil, it is important to compare costs. But is the cost of the product going to make a difference in the quality of CBD that you receive? And if it does matter, how are you going to calculate the CBD oil prices?

The first thing to consider is whether you are purchasing true CBD oil or if you are purchasing mostly a carrier oil. Since CBD is going to be considered an active ingredient, the volume of the oil is not going to matter quite as much, but the percentage of CBD that the oil contains will. This is where bigger is not always better. It will do you no good to get a huge bottle of oil that has almost no CBD inside it, even if it is cheaper than other options. But how do you calculate and compare the costs?

Before we go further here, it is important to remember that the price of the oil is not the only thing to consider. You should also look at the quality, where it comes from, whether it was extracted using good practices, and how reliable the oil is.

Something that you should consider is the bioavailability of the product to help you get the best deal. To keep it simple, bioavailability is the strength of the compound when it reaches the site of physiological activity. This is a major factor of how beneficial the CBD product is overall. There are a lot of forms that

CBD can be produced in, from ointments, pastes, and suppositories, all with different ways of being administered.

Not only is the percentage of CBD inside the product important when it comes to how much it will cost, but it is also important to consider how strong the product will be when it reaches the place in the body where it is most needed. You can also consider delivery time, which is going to depend on the other ingredients inside the product, as well as the form and the method you work with to administer the oil.

While all the methods can be effective, the most bioavailable method for taking CBD will be the suppository form. Since this is not a method most people prefer, you will have to consider the bioavailability when picking out one of the other methods.

Now it is time to figure out the price of the CBD. First, take a look at the product and see how many milligrams of CBD it contains. If you see that the CBD content is on the label in the form of a percentage, use some calculations to figure the volume. Simply multiply by the percentage to find out how many milligrams of CBD are inside the bottle.

The next question is: How much does the pure CBD oil cost? Let's say you are thinking about purchasing a bottle of hemp oil that is 10ml but contains 300mg of CBD. If this bottle costs $32, divide this by the 300 to determine the price you are paying per milligram of CBD. This result is $0.11 per milligram for a 3 percent CBD product.

A $194, 10 ml bottle of hemp oil contains 1500 mg of CBD. The price is $0.13 per milligram of CBD.

While the second product contains more CBD, the cost per milligram is higher, so it is not the best deal for you. You can use these calculations to determine if you are getting a good deal. A bigger bottle is not necessarily a better bottle.

Chapter 9: Legal Aspects to Consider

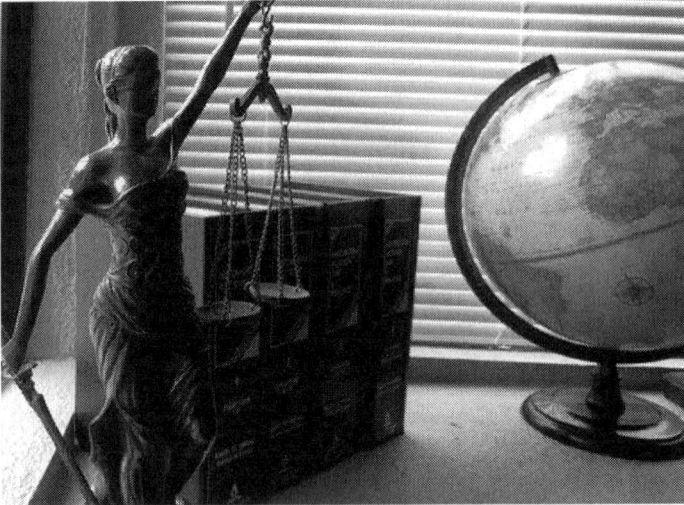

While there are a lot of health benefits of using CBD oil, there are still a lot of questions about whether it is legal to use it or not. This is a grey area of the law. While this oil is not made from the same part of the cannabis plant as marijuana, the United States, the United Kingdom, and other western countries do not differentiate between the different parts of the cannabis plant. All products are technically considered illegal.

So, does this mean that when you sell or purchase CBD oil, you are doing something that is illegal?

For years, the business of CBD oil survived on the ambiguity of the Federal Controlled Substances Act and its definition of marijuana. This act does not include the plant's mature stalks in its definition of "marijuana". These mature stalks are the part of the cannabis plant used to make hemp. Hemp is not prohibited under this Controlled Substances Act. Since non-psychoactive CBD oil is made out of hemp, many manufacturers and users were able to get around the rules of the Controlled Substances Act and could technically sell the product, even in areas where marijuana is illegal.

This ambiguity was then enlarged more with the passage of the 2014 Farm Bill. This bill allowed some cultivation of hemp with THC levels below 0.3 percent. Since this is the level of most CBD oils, many manufacturers and suppliers of CBD could sell the oil under the law's provisions.

But even though these two bills seem to make CBD oil legal, other complications come into play. Since marijuana is a controlled substance and is illegal throughout most of the United States, sale of any part of the cannabis plant is technically illegal.

In 2016, the Drug Enforcement Administration decided to address the issues with CBD and its products to avoid the technicalities and help people know where they stood on these products. It released regulations that made it virtually impossible for suppliers to work around the definition of marijuana as found in the Controlled Substances Act.

With this new rule, there is a new Controlled Substances Code Number that includes information on marijuana extract that extends classification to extracts with one or more cannabinoids from any plant of the genus *Cannabis*. Since CBD is a cannabinoid, and hemp is a plant from the genus *Cannabis*, the new rule applies to most CBD products that are sold online and in shops.

Furthermore, the DEA confirmed that, "for practical purposes, all extracts that contain CBD will also contain at least small amounts of other cannabinoids. However, if it were possible to produce from the cannabis plant an extract that contained only CBD... such an abstract would fall within the new drug code 7350." The new DEA directive helps the Agency comply with the UN Convention on Narcotic Drugs and ensures that suppliers cannot dance around some of the loopholes in the previous bills.

What is this going to mean for suppliers and sellers of CBD extracts either online or in states that do not have more progressive cannabis laws? While there are a lot of flowery words around the issue, the DEA now explicitly considers CBD oil illegal under the Controlled Substances Act, just like other illicit cannabis products. The Agency is also working to enhance its ability to track CBD and enforce its interpretation of the law.

While this may seem like a blow to the industry, it is most likely that CBD merchants were always on the wrong side, or at least in the gray area, when it comes to the DEA. This is because the CBD extracts used in CBD oil always contain other types of cannabinoids. Currently, the oil cannot be produced absent of other types of cannabinoids. This issue has always been recognized, but now the DEA is able (and eager) to enforce the law on sellers if they are caught.

While the DEA is hardening its laws about CBD oil, there are still many sellers who can sell the product. Many of these are located in areas where cannabis is legal, so they are not going against the law. However, if you live in an area where cannabis and marijuana are illegal, you could be in trouble if you are caught with the substance.

There are a lot of good benefits of CBD and more people are starting to see them. However, cannabis products are still technically illegal in some States. And until the laws are changed, you need to realize you could face issues when you obtain these kinds of products, especially if you live in a state where the cannabis is illegal. The UK has changed its view on CBD and will now allow doctors to prescribe CBD (cannabidiol) for medical uses provided the THC content is no more than 0.2% and that the THC cannot be separated from the CBD. Additionally, recreational cannabis use is still illegal in most countries. True CBD oil with trace amounts of THC is legal in the UK and in some states, however you should still exercise caution when purchasing. In my opinion the prohibition of cannabis will eventually come to an end and governments will allow (and tax) cannabis in the same way as alcohol and nicotine products.

If you need CBD to help with a medical problem, you should consider talking to your doctor. This will allow you to get a prescription to use the oil legally. There are provisions in most states allowing you to obtain CBD oil if you need it for medical purposes.

And, if you are in a state where cannabis is legal, make sure you are purchasing the product from someone in a state where it is legal. Make sure that you either have a doctor's note or that you live in an area where it is legal to make sure you avoid issues with the law.

Chapter 10: CBD Oil and Your Pets

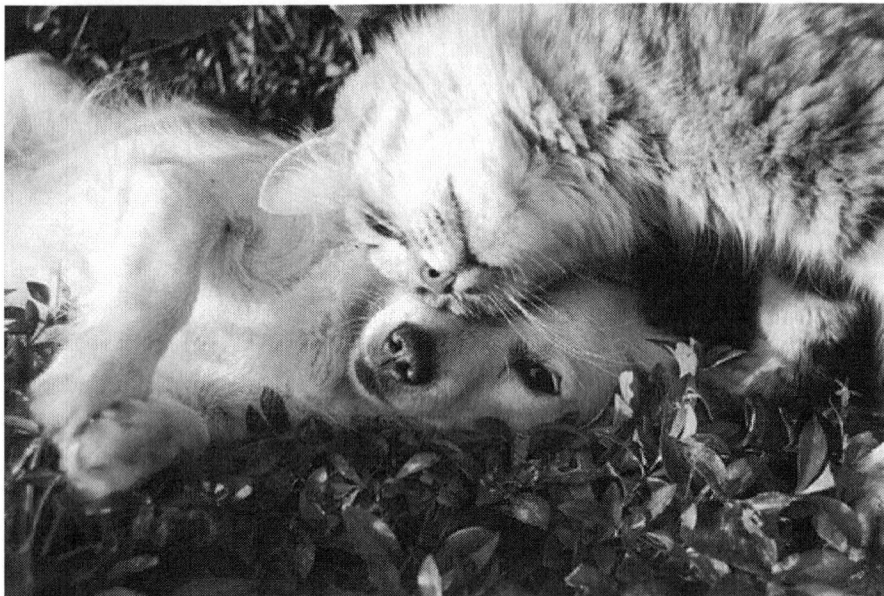

Not only are you able to use CBD oil to improve your own health, it can also be used to improve the health of your pets. CBD oil is just as effective on your pet as it can be on human beings and there are a ton of great health benefits that come from using it. All mammals can use CBD oil, you just need to make sure that you follow the right dosage (based on size) to ensure that they are able to see the best benefits. Let's take a look at how CBD oil can be used on your pets and some of the great health benefits they will receive when they start using this product.

What can CBD oil treat in pets?

You will be amazed at how many different things CBD oil is able to do to help your pet. While most pet owners use different medications to help their pets feel better and deal with a variety of common ailments, they can't treat everything. And they often come with a lot of harmful side effects. This makes it a great option, especially if other treatments do not work.

Benefits include:

- Reducing anxiety: Anxiety can be a tough disorder to deal with. Human beings are able to discuss their feelings and emotions, but your pet is not able to handle anxiety in this way. When the anxiety gets severe enough, it can result in destructive behaviors like scratching, urinating indoors, chewing, and barking. CBD relaxes your pets, so they can stay calm and not react a negative way. This could be beneficial for animals who are nervous and perhaps made more uncomfortable with loud noises, e.g. roadworks or fireworks.

- Chronic pain relief: When your pet is dealing chronic pain, there are very few options on the market. CBD oil helps keep your pet comfortable because it targets inflammation in the joints. It could also help with dental problems. Not only does it help reduce the amount of pain felt, but it can also help the healing process.

- Loss of appetite: If your pet has trouble eating or has pain and nausea that makes it hard to eat, CBD could do the trick. There are treat options on the market that can provide relief for your pet.

- Seizures: Not only can cannabis help human beings who suffer from seizures, your pet can benefit as well. CBD oil for pets can be used to manage seizures and can reduce their occurrence. This is a huge relief for the pet and for the pet owner, and it will improve your pet's quality of life.

- Aggressive behavior: There are a lot of reasons why your pet may show aggressive behavior. With the help of CBD, you can help calm your pet. It can even help with some stress disorders that your pet experiences, making them healthier and happier.

- IBS: CBD can be used to help treat irritable bowel syndrome in your pet. It has anti-inflammatory properties, so it will make your pet more comfortable. It could help eliminate the disease altogether.

- Glaucoma: Dogs and other animals who are dealing with glaucoma have used CBD. Ingesting CBD sublingually reduces the pressure in the eye. More studies need to be done to see whether this pressure reduction is permanent, but the treatment does provide some temporary relief.

- Heart health: There are many health benefits that come from using CBD. The most important one is that CBD improves cardiac function in dogs suffering from arrhythmia. This can help to reduce the incidences of cardiac events and improves blood flow to most of the major organs.

- Bone health: CBD can also benefit animals that have broken a bone or are dealing with severe osteoporosis. Studies demonstrate how using CBD can stimulate new bone growth while also strengthening bones that are damaged through osteoporosis. Also there are pain killing and anti-inflammatory properties to CBD which makes it even more ideal.

- Brain: CBD is a powerful neuro-protectant, meaning that it works to protect the nerve cells from issues with impairment, degeneration, and damage. When it is administered after a neurological event or as ongoing treatment for those who have a high likelihood of a neurological event, CBD can help protect the brain from any damage and will reduce the likelihood of a recurrence.

- Diabetes: CBD can help to regulate blood sugar levels and can mitigate the symptoms of diabetes. When it is used correctly, it can reduce damage in the pancreas and, in type 2 diabetes, it can help to improve sensitivity to insulin.

- Immune system: CBD can help with auto-immune illnesses in your pet. It has been effective at regulating the overactive immune system in pets and could reduce the damage that this has on the nature structures and functions of the body.

- Infections: There are several types of bacterial growth that can be slowed down by the use of CBD. Sometimes, it can help to kill bacteria fully. It has been effective in dealing with some medication-resistant bacterial strains.

- Sleep: Dogs with canine cognitive dysfunction were able to enjoy improved sleep patterns by taking CBD oil. This helped them to sleep during the night because it induced drowsiness.

- Psoriasis: While it is rare, your pet could suffer from psoriasis, and CBD can help to treat this disease.

- Muscle relaxant: CBD can help treat not only muscle spasms, but it also works to help with conditions that cause the muscles of your pet to tighten up. It helps them to relax, so that your pet is not so stiff and sore.

- Blood flow: There are numerous reasons that your pet could be suffering from poor blood flow including problems with the valves of their heart and heartworms. The CBD can work to improve circulation and can reduce some of the complications that accompany bad blood flow.

Which pets can use CBD oil?

Almost every animal will be able to benefit from CBD oil. The most common animals to use CBD include cats and dogs, but other mammals can enjoy it as well.

If you are using the CBD on larger animals, it is especially important to talk to your vet before starting this treatment. You will need to give larger doses to these animals because of their size and your vet can make sure you are using it properly and in the right dosage.

What dosage is right for my pet?

Proper dosage is crucial and based on the animal's weight. Initially, it is best to try about 1-5 mg per every 10 pounds of body weight. As always, start with the lowest amount and then increase if needed.

For most cats, you are fine giving them 1mg due to their relatively light weight. For heavier dogs, follow the weight related guidelines. Always monitor how your pet reacts and if there are any major side effects. If there are going to be any changes, these will occur within an hour. If you do not see any changes, then it is time to increase the dosage.

If you are using the CBD for pain relief, the treatment should be given about once every eight hours. If you are using it to correct unwanted behavior in your animal, two times a day is best. Of course, you may need to do more than one treatment in order to see the improvement you seek.

There is very little risk to overdosing your pet with pure CBD, however if the CBD treatment has trace amounts of THC, make sure to monitor your pet to see any signs of toxicity. Watch them for any signs that they are suffering from a high. This may include your pet having trouble eating, walking, or standing.

CBD can be very helpful to animals. If your pet is dealing with a debilitating ailment, and you want to try a method without harmful side effects, CBD oil may be the answer. Talk to your vet before starting any treatment. Most vets are familiar with how CBD oil influences animals and they will be able to discuss usage and best practices with you.

Chapter 11: Success Stories from Those Who Used CBD Oil

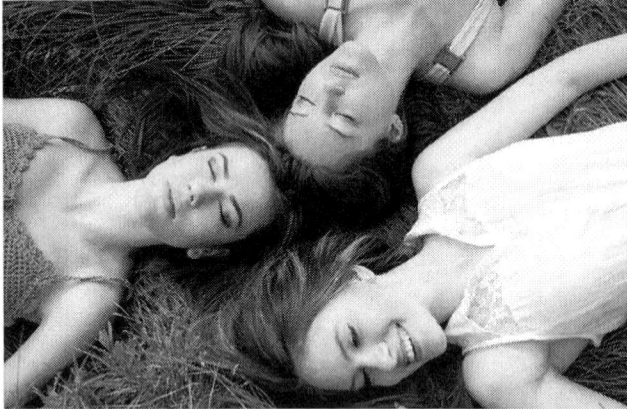

There are a lot of people who have relied on CBD oil to help them feel better. Some may have been on traditional medications and found that they did not work well. Others wanted to find an all-natural treatment. Here are some of the success stories from CBD oil and from those who were finally able to get some relief by using this product.

- Patient 1: I dealt with chronic headaches that were caused from a traumatic brain injury and a concussion about five years ago. I tried a few other products, and nothing worked. I then decided to try CBD and in just a few weeks, I was pressure and pain free. This was the first time since my accident. In addition, it was also able to help with my mild anxiety that was caused by some hormonal changes after the accident. It also makes it easier for me to focus than ever before.

- Patient 2: I suffer from multiple sclerosis. I have multiple symptoms of MS including insomnia, spasms, fatigue, and headaches. After trying several brands and experimenting with the dosage, I finally found a good night time and morning oil to use. Since I started with CBD, I have been able to stop taking my other prescription medications, other than my daily MS medication. Even without these medications, I feel so much better than I have in a long time. And I also have energy I never knew I had!

- Patient 3: I have suffered two strokes in the past four years. After these occurred, I was diagnosed with rheumatoid arthritis. I was often depressed and down in the dumps. I was also lethargic and short-tempered. And the pain I felt from the arthritis meant that it was difficult doing even the smallest tasks. No one wants to live that way. My doctors and specialists gave me lots of drugs, but they never really helped me to feel better. One day, my son called to tell me what he had heard about CBD oil. A few months ago, I decided to start using it. I used one drop, three times a day for a few weeks. Then I increased to two drops of green, two times a day and then two drops of gold at night. I feel a lot better and can enjoy life again.

- Patient 4: For the last 22 years, I have been on disability. I was in so much pain that all I could think about was how to get rid of the pain. As soon as I found the CBD oil, it changed my life. I went down from high pain to mid pain and since I was finally able to get up and move, I started to lose weight. This has helped me to enjoy my life more than ever.

- Patient 5: I suffered from headaches all the time, which usually turned into migraines. My husband fell ill a few years ago, which increased my depression and anxiety. It was hard for me to maintain a happy attitude when I was in so much pain and suffering from depression. Someone from his support group had seen success with CBD oil, so I looked it up and realized it might help me, too. I experimented a bit with the dosage and found taking one drop, three times a day helped to make the headaches go away. It also helped my anxiety diminish and I am slowly weaning off the anti-depressants.

- Patient 6: Two-and-a-half years ago, I was diagnosed with a disease called CVID. I require immunoglobulin infusions for the rest of my life. About nine months after that, I was diagnosed with chronic lymphocytic leukemia. This is all on top of bad migraines for 35 years and fibromyalgia for 25 years. I needed a lot of medications and often felt like I was not functioning well at all. It was at this time I decided to give CBD oil a try. I hoped it would give me some relief from the pain. Within just a few weeks, I got relief from all of the pain I had, including migraines, bones, fibromyalgia, and back. After working up to a dose that seemed the best for me, I was able to reduce the pain meds by 75 percent. I still suffer from the diseases, but CBD oil has changed things in a way that allows me to function better.

- Patient 7: CBD has helped me to deal with my fibromyalgia pain. After dealing with this disease for the past 20+ years, it had gotten so bad that I qualified for disability. I spent a lot of time in bed because of the pain, and I suffered from anxiety and depression. I started taking CBD 7 months ago and my body seemed to respond right away. I have less pain and am able to get more done through the day.

- Patient 8: I have dealt with anxiety for most of my life, and as I've grown older, the panic attacks have worsened. Since I have always been health-conscious, I figured that working out and eating right would help take care of it. This did not happen. I decided that 2018 would be the year for me to take care of my mental health, and that is when I came across CBD oil. Since I've started taking it, I have seen a big improvement and have only dealt with one panic attack over the past two months. It has helped me to realize what normal is supposed to feel like.

- Patient 9: I am dealing with severe osteoarthritis, spondylolisthesis, and scoliosis of the spine. All the vertebrae in the back have been fused from T4 down. These fusions were from failed back surgeries, so I have been dealing with chronic pain. CBD oil has helped reduce the pain and allowed me to decrease the use of Norco. I still have some pain, but I feel better and I do not have to worry about being impaired by excessive opioid use.

- Patient 10: I am dealing with an autoimmune disease known as polymyalgia rheumatica. This condition effects the muscles in the hips, shoulders, and neck. I have suffered from chronic inflammation pain for the past ten months and was told that I had to take prednisone to take away the pain. I wanted to find more natural relief. I started taking CBD oil and after just three days, I could feel that my joints were loosening up. Four months later, I still have a bit of discomfort in my shoulders, but I have my life back.

- Patient 11: I suffer from many different diseases. These include anxiety, nausea, migraines, chronic pain, bipolar depression, PTSD, and fibromyalgia pain. My pain was a 10 all day long before I took CBD oil. I never took pain medications because I don't have a tolerance for them, and the few I took for fibromyalgia didn't work and gave a lot of bad side effects. I started using about 350mg of CBD oil for a month. I noticed right away that it helped to calm my anxiety. After one month, I do not feel as nauseous and the pain is less intense. I plan to adjust the dosage to see if it helps out even more with some of my disorders.

- Patient 12: Many people in my family have arthritis, fibromyalgia, and lupus. I do as well. The pain got really bad last year and made my sleeping problems worse. I wasn't able to walk after I finished work and did not have any energy to do anything. It was at this time that I heard about CBD oil and I tried it out. I am now able to walk around stores, get to sleep, spend more time with my kids and just live life. And this is after only a week of being on it!

Chapter 12: What Will the Future Bring

As more people learn about CBD oil and all the benefits that come from using it, it is likely that the public perception about it will change. And as the public perception changes, it is even more likely that many states, and eventually the national government, will start to change the current laws about the oil and allow everyone to use it legally.

This will make a big difference in the future of cannabis and its products. First, once it becomes legal, the stigma that surrounds cannabis will be lifted. People will stop thinking about it as such a bad thing, and there will be less judgment against those who decide to use the plant for their health and general well-being.

When cannabis becomes legal, it will be easier to get CBD and CBD products. More people will be willing to sell it since they won't get in trouble with the authorities. This offers more options and a lot of benefits to the consumer.

This is becoming a very popular market. With more people selling CBD, the market will naturally become more competitive. Right now, there are a limited number of distributors of CBD oil because the product is considered illegal in many countries. Many sellers can only sell their products online or in the places where it is allowed and legal in their country. These distributors are able to set the price wherever they want, which can end up being higher than what some people can afford.

As more distributors get into the market, the price will naturally go down. There is more competition, so sellers are less likely to hike up the price to something that is outrageous just because they can. This will make it easier for individuals to get the CBD oil at an affordable price.

Once cannabis finally becomes legal, perhaps the industry will be subject to stricter regulations. In some cases, this may be a bad thing because regulation may impose a lot of harsh rules. Still making cannabis available as a medication can only be seen as something positive. Currently, it is really hard to know if the CBD oil you are getting is good or if the sellers have added stuff to the mix that could reduce its potency. With regulations in place, "cutting" would no longer be a problem because all distributors would need to follow the set guidelines before they were allowed to sell.

In addition, when cannabis and CBD oil are legal, more studies can be done on the health benefits of taking this product. Right now, limited numbers of legal consumers mean limited opportunities for study. If the product were legal, more individuals would start taking it, and it would be easier for researchers to gather information. Based on the scientific studies that we have so far, this can only mean good things for showing how much CBD oil can benefit your health.

And the best part of all, if cannabis and CBD oil became legal, it would mean that more people would have access to an all-natural and safe remedy for many of their common ailments. For those who may have tried other costly treatments (with bad side effects or limited effectiveness), legalizing the product may finally provide the answer they seek.

Bonus Chapter 1: Medical Marijuana Discussed

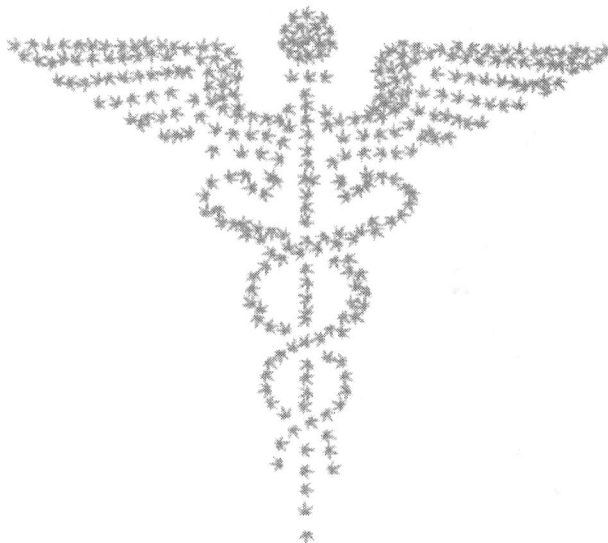

Medical marijuana is any part of the cannabis plant used to help treat health problems. While some varieties contain more THC and can give the user a bit of a high, the primary use of medical marijuana is to cure a disease or provide relief for the sufferer. Most of the marijuana that is legally sold as medicine will have the same ingredients as what is found in the kind used for pleasure. However, there are some types of medical marijuana that have been developed with fewer chemicals that can cause the high.

The marijuana plant will have multiple chemicals, or cannabinoids, and as we have looked at the two main ones are CBD and THC. Research shows how CBD can be used for some health issues. Most medical marijuana types contain higher levels of this chemical.

People who smoke medical marijuana will begin to feel its effects almost right away. If you eat it though, it can take closer to two or sometimes up to three hours to feel the effects. When you smoke it, the THC goes from the lungs to the bloodstream almost instantly. It then causes the brain cells to release dopamine, which makes you feel good and reduces the pain that you feel.

The flowers or buds in the cannabis plant can be dried, ground then smoked either in a joint with tobacco and rolled with cigarette papers, or in a pipe or a vaporizer. Smoking cannabis in this manner will allow the user to consume all of the compounds found in cannabis including a relatively high amount of THC. Recreational marijuana use can make a person feel quite relaxed and expand the senses. Sensations of touch and feel, taste and sound are enhanced. Listening to music can take on an added depth and the flavors in foods taste more intense. This 'high' can open up your mind to new concepts and ideas but can also make the user a bit giddy and giggly at times. These effects can last several hours. There can be downsides though.

Aside from the legal implications, smoking too much weed can make some people a bit irritable, confused or even slightly paranoid. A heavy user might become lethargic with a loss of drive and confidence and can appear a bit unkempt or tired. Long term there could be more serious mental implications. A heavy cannabis smoker can sometimes favor to be solitary rather than going out socializing. Of course, everyone is different, and the effects will vary.

Over the long term, smoking too much marijuana with a high THC content may trigger an underlying mental illness that might otherwise go undetected. Paranoia or anxiety could develop in a person who's already susceptible to these conditions. If such symptoms appear, it is advisable to stop smoking completely. Most people should return to full health within a short time.

Is smoking cannabis recreationally a gate way to harder drugs? It may be with people with addictive personalities. Such individuals could, in time, progress from smoking cigarettes to drinking alcohol to smoking weed to trying other drugs and so on. And while cannabis (along with just about any other substance) can become addictive, the average person who sometimes uses cannabis recreationally will not automatically be dragged to a life of drug-fueled mayhem; rather they will use it occasionally just like they would with alcohol.

Medical marijuana can be used for many different types of health issues. It can help with loss of appetite, nausea, and can ease pain. It can also help with symptoms of multiple sclerosis and with epilepsy.

While there are a lot of great benefits that come with medical marijuana, it is important to get a prescription from your doctor before you decide to use it. There are some concerns about the legality of medical marijuana and CBD oil, and it is always better to get things covered. This helps you to avoid problems while also getting the health benefits from this product.

Are there any FDA approved marijuana medications?

Right now, there are two medications containing THC that are approved by the FDA. These drugs are called dronabinol and nabilone. They are used in treating nausea that is caused by chemotherapy and they increase appetite in patients who are dealing with extreme weight loss from cancer or AIDS.

These two medications were approved due to the recent research conducted on marijuana and its extracts. Hopefully, research will continue, and more medications will be approved in the future.

In addition, Canada, the United Kingdom, and several other European countries have recently approved nabiximols. This is a mouth spray that contains CBD and THC. It is used to help out with muscle control problems caused by MS. Right now, nabiximols are not approved by the FDA, but since other western countries have approved it, and since the FDA has started to approve medications that contain THC, it is possible this medication will be approved for use in the United States soon.

Points to remember

- The term "medical marijuana" refers to treating symptoms of a condition or illness with the whole, unprocessed marijuana plant or some of its basic extracts.

- The FDA has not approved or even recognized marijuana as a medicine.

- However, scientific study of the chemicals found in marijuana, known as cannabinoids, has led to two FDA-approved medications, dronabinol and nabilone. These are used to boost appetite and treat nausea.

- Currently, the two main cannabinoids from the marijuana plant that are of interest for medical treatment are CBD and THC.

- The body also produces the cannabinoid chemicals on its own. Sometimes these get blocked and are not able to work efficiently.

- Scientists and researchers are still conducting preclinical and clinical trials concerning marijuana and its extracts to treat symptoms of illness and some other conditions.

Bonus Chapter 2: Marijuana Recipes

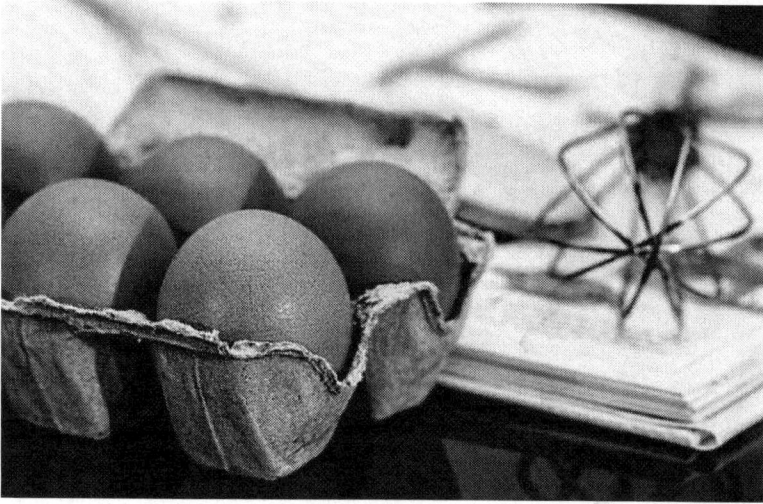

For some people, consuming the CBD oil on its own can be hard. You may not want to wait for it to be absorbed by holding it in your mouth, or you may not like the flavor. If this is the case for you, or you are just looking for a better and tastier way to take your oil, then going with marijuana edibles can be the right choice. This chapter shows you a few different recipes to make your own marijuana edibles at home.

Before we start on these recipes though, it's important to reemphasize the difference between cannabis and medical marijuana. Marijuana is a cannabis plant that is harvested in a way to preserve its euphoric psychoactive properties. The stalks and the fibers are not used commercially. These plants are cultivated to get the flowers from the plant.

To help farmers get the maximum levels of THC in the marijuana plant, it's grown inside so that they can monitor the humidity, temperature, and light. The male plants are removed to help keep the female plants from being fertilized. If the female is fertilized, it will lower the concentration of THC.

Medical marijuana or Medical Cannabis is a form of this plant used to help with medical conditions. Often the levels of THC will be lower, but the intended effect is to help cure a medical condition. There will still be levels of THC in the medical marijuana, but often those are helpful to keep the anxiety and stress levels of the patient down during treatment.

With CBD oil, you are receiving the seeds and the stalks from the cannabis plant. Its seeds and stalks can be used to produce many products such as plastic composites, building materials, nutritional supplements, food, and medicines.

Because it will thrive under some natural conditions, CBD is grown outside, with the female and male plants grown together to help encourage pollination and seed production. The hemp plant will grow sturdy and strong.

As long as the THC content is below 0.3 percent, it is usually legal to consume. It can be used for medicinal purposes as well. But since the THC levels are lower, it doesn't require a doctor's note in order to consume.

In the recipes below, we are talking about CBD oil, not about medical marijuana. You can cook with medical marijuana/cannabis as well however this should be done with some caution. You would need to be sure of the exact amount and type of THC before consuming as the effects will vary depending of the quantity and strength of THC present in medical marijuana. If you need medical marijuana for a medical condition, then you can substitute. But CBD oil is often seen more beneficial for your health and these recipes can make consuming the oil tastier than ever before.

Breakfasts

Banana Bread

Ingredients:
1 egg
2 Tbsp. honey
¼ c. cannabis butter
¼ c. buttermilk
1 ½ c. mashed bananas
½ tsp. nutmeg
½ tsp. baking soda
½ tsp. baking powder
½ tsp. salt
¼ c. packed brown sugar
¼ c. sugar
½ c. whole wheat flour
½ c. all-purpose flour
Cooking spray
1 tsp. vanilla

Directions
1. Turn on the oven to 350 degrees. Take out 7 mini-loaf pans and coat them with some cooking spray.
2. Take out a bowl and combine both the flours with the nutmeg, baking soda, baking powder, salt, brown sugar, and sugar.
3. In a second bowl, combine the vanilla, egg, honey, butter, buttermilk, and bananas. Use a mixer to beat these together well.
4. Add the dry ingredients into a bowl and then mix to make combined. Pour this into the loaf pans, just slightly over half full.
5. Add these to the oven and let them bake for 20 minutes, or until the bread is done. Allow them some time to cool

on a wire rack for a few minutes before taking out of the pan. Cool a bit longer before serving or storing.

Carrot and Raisin Muffins

Ingredients:
2 tsp. pumpkin pie spice
1 Tbsp. baking powder
1/3 c. packed brown sugar
1 ½ c. all-purpose flour
1 ½ c. raisin bran cereal
2 Tsp. orange zest, grated
1 egg
¼ c. vegetable oil
¼ c. cannabis vegetable oil
1 c. carrots, shredded
1 c. milk
¾ c. walnuts, chopped
1 c. raisins
½ tsp. salt

Directions:
1. Turn on the oven to 374 degrees. Take out 12 muffin cups and add some paper liners inside.
2. In a bowl, whisk together the orange zest, egg, vegetable oil, cannabis oil, carrots, and milk.
3. In a second bowl, mix together the salt, pumpkin pie spice, baking powder, brown sugar, sugar, flour, and bran flakes.
4. Add the wet ingredients in with the dry ones and then stir to moisten the flour. Stir in the raisins and walnuts.
5. Spoon this into the muffin cups, leaving a little bit of room on the top.
6. Bake these muffins for 25 minutes. Serve them either warm or wait until they have time to cool down first.

Baby Pancakes

Ingredients:
2 Tbsp. confectioners' sugar
Juice from half a lemon
¼ c. butter
1/8 tsp. nutmeg
½ tsp. salt
1 Tbsp. sugar
1 Tbsp. cannabis milk
3 eggs
¾ c. flour
¾ c. milk

Directions
1. Heat up the oven to 425 degrees. Take out a bowl and combine the sugar, cannabis milk, eggs, flour, milk nutmeg, and salt. Stir until there are no lumps.
2. Take out a cast iron skillet and melt the butter over medium heat. When the butter is melted, pour the batter into the pan and then the skillet over to the oven.
3. Bake this mixture for 20 minutes so the pancake has time to become golden brown and puffed.
4. Turn the temperature of the oven down to 300 degrees. Bake this for another 5 minutes before taking the pancake out of the oven.
5. Sprinkle on the sugar and lemon juice before serving.

Bacon, Cheese, and Egg Quiches

Ingredients:
¼ tsp. pepper
¼ tsp. salt
¼ c. cannabis half and half
½ c. half and half
2 eggs

¾ c. Cheddar cheese
½ c. bacon bits, cooked
3 Tbsp. milk
2 Tbsp. vegetable shortening
2 Tbsp. butter
¾ c. flour
Cooking spray

Directions:
1. Turn on the oven to 375 degrees. Grease the muffin cups with some cooking spray.
2. Work on the crust first. Add the shortening, butter, and flour to your food processor and pulse it for 10 times to help cut the butter inside the flour until it is combined.
3. Place this mixture over to a bowl and then stir in the milk so that it holds the dough together. Make it into a bowl and then flatten it into a disc. Wrap this in some plastic wrap and put in the fridge for a minimum of 30 minutes.
4. Flour a clean surface and use a rolling pin to roll out the crust. Take a 2 ½ inch cookie cutter and make 24 circles. Press these into the muffin cups.
5. Sprinkle some bacon bits into the cup and top with some shredded cheese.
6. Take out a bowl and whisk together the pepper, salt, cannabis half and half, half and half, and the eggs. Pour this into each of the muffin cups until filled.
7. Place this into the oven and bake for 40 minutes or until the quiches have time to set. Allow to cool before serving.

Main Meals

Cheesy Fettuccini

Ingredients:
1 c. mozzarella cheese

¾ c. Parmesan cheese
1 tsp. pepper
Salt
2 c. half and half
1 Tbsp. garlic, minced
2 Tbsp. cannabis butter
½ c. and 2 Tbsp. butter
1 ½ lbs. fettuccine

Directions:
1. Use the directions on the package to cook the fettuccine. Drain and set to the side.
2. Take out a pan and melt the cannabis butter and better. Add the garlic and stir for 30 seconds before adding in the pepper, salt, and half and half.
3. Bring this to a simmer, stirring often to prevent it from boiling over. When ready, stir in the Parmesan and cook for another 5 minutes.
4. After this time, stir in the mozzarella and cook until this melts as well. Take the pan from the heat and use an immersion blender to get the sauce smooth.
5. Pour this over the prepared pasta and serve.

Shrimp Creole

Ingredients

1/8 tsp. cayenne pepper
1 bay leaf
1 Tbsp. cannabis oil
2 Tbsp. chopped parsley
1 c. chicken stock
1 can tomatoes, crushed
2 tsp. minced garlic
1 diced celery rib
½ diced green bell pepper

½ diced onion
2 Tbsp. flour
1 Tbsp. olive oil
1 Tbsp. butter
Cooked rice
1 lb. peeled shrimp
Salt

Directions:
1. In a skillet, melt the better and the olive oil. Whisk in the flour and cook until a light roux forms. This will take about 4 minutes.
2. Add in the celery, bell pepper, and onion and stir to combine until the vegetables are soft, about 4 minutes.
3. Stir in the garlic and cook for another minute. After that time, stir in the tomatoes with their juices, the salt, cayenne, bay leaf, cannabis oil, parsley, and stock.
4. Increase the heat to bring this to a boil and then reduce to a simmer to cook for 15 minutes.
5. Add in the shrimp, stirring to combine, and cook another 5 minutes until the shrimp is done. Remove the bay leaf and serve over rice.

Honey Lime Chicken

Ingredients:
2 c. cooked rice
Scallions
2 tsp. toasted sesame seeds
½ tsp. sesame oil
1 tsp. ginger
1 tsp. sriracha hot sauce
2 Tbsp. lime juice
2 Tbsp. cannabis honey
6 Tbsp. honey

½ c. light soy sauce
Pepper
Salt
1 chicken, sliced into 8 pieces

Directions:
1. Turn on the grill to 375 degrees. Use the pepper and salt to season the chicken pieces. Cook on the grill until cooked through.
2. While your chicken cooks, prepare the glaze. Take out a pan and combine the rest of the ingredients, except the rice.
3. Heat over the stove, stirring until it starts to bubble. Reduce the heat and cook until it is thick, another three minutes.
4. Place the chicken into a bowl and toss to coat with the glass. Garnish and serve over rice.

Snacks and Desserts

Caramel Corn

Ingredients:
1 tsp. vanilla
¾ tsp. baking soda
2 tsp. salt
¼ c. honey
1 c. dark brown sugar
1 Tbsp. cannabis butter
1/3 c. butter
12 c. popped popcorn, plain

Directions;
1. Preheat the oven to 225 degrees. Take out two baking sheets and line with parchment paper.

2. Place your popcorn in a bowl. Bring out a pan and melt the cannabis butter and butter. Stir in with the salt, honey, and brown sugar. Stir this on the stove until the mixture starts to boil.
3. Lower the heat to a simmer. Cook for about 90 seconds. Take the pan from the heat and add in the vanilla and baking soda. Pour over the popcorn and toss to coat before it hardens.
4. Spread this onto the baking sheets and put into the oven. Bake for 15 minutes.
5. Take out of the oven at this time and stir around the popcorn to break up the pieces. Allow to cook for another 15 minutes.

Chocolate Chip Cookies

Ingredients:
1 c. chocolate chips
½ tsp. salt
½ tsp. baking soda
1 1/8 c. flour
1 egg
1 tsp. vanilla
¼ c. butter
¼ c. cannabis butter
2/3 c. brown sugar
2/3 c. sugar

Directions:
1. Turn the oven on to 375 degrees. While that is heating up, bring out a bowl and beat the vanilla, butter, cannabis butter, brown sugar, and sugar together until creamy. Beat in the egg next.
2. In a second bowl, stir together the salt, baking soda, and flour. When those are combined, beat them into the butter mixture along with the chocolate chips.

3. Drop some of the cookie dough onto baking sheets and then place into the oven to bake.
4. After 15 minutes, take the cookies out of the oven and serve warm.

Brownies

Ingredients:
¾ c. macadamia nuts
½ tsp. vanilla
3 eggs
1 c. brown sugar
4 ½ oz. chocolate
¼ c. cannabis coconut oil
1/3 c. coconut oil
¾ tsp. salt
2 Tbsp. cocoa powder
¾ c. flour

Directions:
1. Turn on the oven to 350 degrees. Bring out a bowl and combine the salt, cocoa powder, and flour.
2. In a pan, melt the chocolate, cannabis coconut oil, and coconut oil together over a low heat. When these are melted, set aside and let cool for five minutes.
3. After that time, stir in the brown sugar along with the vanilla and the egg. Add in the flour mixture and the nuts.
4. When this is ready, pour onto some prepared baking pans and put into the oven. Bake for 30 minutes until they are done. Take out of the oven and allow to cool before serving.

Cannabis Pantry Items

Cannabis butter

Ingredients:
½ oz. crumbed decarboxylated cannabis
1 ¼ c. butter

Directions:
1. Take out the slow cooker and add the butter and cannabis inside.
2. Place the lid on top and cook on low for 4 to 6 hours. Use right away or store.

Cannabis oil

Ingredients:
½ oz. crumbled decarboxylated cannabis
1 ¼ c. edible oil (your choice)

Directions:
1. Add the cannabis and the oil to the top of a double boiler. Let it cook over some simmering water for 4 hours.
2. Make sure to check the water level so that you can add more when needed.
3. Store or use right away.

Cannabis cream or milk

Ingredients:
½ oz. crumbled cannabis
1 ¼ c. heavy cream or whole milk

Directions:
1. Bring a pan of water to a simmer and place a towel in the bottom of the pan.
2. Put the cream or milk along with the cannabis into a Mason jar and cover with a lid.

3. Add the jar to the towel in the simmering water and let it go for 90 minutes.
4. Make sure to check the water levels on a regular basis and add in some more if needed. You can also stir the milk.

Beauty Products with CBD Oil

Body Lotion

Ingredients:
.5-gram CBD isolate
2 c. olive oil
Favorite essential oil (4 drops)

Directions:
1. Mix the three ingredients together so that the CBD isolate can dissolve and get mixed into the solution.
2. Use this on any part of the body that needs some body lotion or that is experiencing pain.
3. If you add in some salt and a little lavender oil, you can make a good body scrub with the oil.

Easy Salve

Ingredients:
1 oz. shea butter
1 oz. beeswax
1 c. CBD infused oil

Directions:
1. Create a double boiler by adding a smaller pot on top of a larger pot with a few inches of water in the bottom.
2. Add in the oil and the beeswax after the oil is at a gentle simmer. Make sure to stir this around often.

3. When the beeswax is almost dissolved, add in the shea butter. Continue to stir until it dissolves completely.
4. Pour this into your chosen containers. Let them set for a few hours to become completely solid.
5. Use when needed.

Anti-Wrinkle Cream

Ingredients:
1 Tbsp. confectioner's cream
1 tsp. vanilla
1 c. cream, heavy
7 g. CBD oil

Directions:
1. Add the oil and the cream to a double boiler. Let the heat be low and simmer these for an hour.
2. After that time, let the cream cool down a bit and then put into a container in the fridge to make cold.
3. Chill your whisk and a large bowl in a freezer for about ten minutes.
4. Take them from the freezer and then add in the prepared cream to it. Whip with a whisk to make some stiff peaks.

Beat in the vanilla and sugar until peaks form. Use this on your skin, rubbing in gently to get the best results.

Dosage Charts

Rough guide for CBD daily dosage.

SEVERITY RANGE	WEIGHT OF PERSON 31-60 lbs	WEIGHT OF PERSON 60-100 lbs	WEIGHT OF PERSON 100-175 lbs	WEIGHT OF PERSON 175-250 lbs
MILD 1	2mg-4mg +	4mg-6mg +	6mg-8mg +	8mg-10mg +
2	4mg-8mg +	6mg-12mg +	8mg-18mg +	12mg-20mg +
MEDIUM 3	8mg-12mg +	12mg-18mg +	18mg-24mg +	22mg-30mg +
4	12mg-18mg +	18mg-24mg +	24mg-32mg +	32mg-40mg +
SEVERE 5	18mg-30mg +	24mg-40mg +	32mg-60mg +	42mg-60mg +

CBD dosage per bottle size

Product Mg	Bottle Size	Drops per bottle	Mg CBD per drop
100 Mg CBD Oil	15 ml	300	.33 mg
300 Mg CBD Oil	15 ml	300	1 mg
600 Mg CBD Oil	15 ml	300	2 mg
900 Mg CBD Oil	15 ml	300	3 mg
1200 Mg CBD Oil	30 ml	600	2 mg
1800 Mg CBD Oil	30 ml	600	3 mg

CBD Chart for Pets.

.

Pets Weight	Dosage
1 – 20 lbs	1 – 2mg/ 2 - 4 drops
21 – 45 lbs	2 – 3mg/ 4 – 6 drops
46 – 74 lbs	3 – 4mg/ 6 -8 drops
75+ lbs	4 – 5mg/ 8 – 10 drops

Appendix: Common Terms to Know

In this book, we spent a lot of time talking about cannabis and CBD oil, as well as how they both work and why they are so good for you. We also brought up a lot of new terms. Here is a quick reference to help you understand if you get stuck during reading or need a reminder:

- Agricultural hemp: The varieties of *Cannabis Sativa L.* The plant contains less than 0.3 percent of THC in the dry weight, and it is grown mostly for industrial purposes. This product is legal for use in the United States and more than 40 other countries.

- *Cannabis Sativa L.*: A species of plant that is found in the genus *Cannabis*. It will refer to both marijuana and agricultural hemp, two completely different plants that are both sub species of cannabis.

- CBD: Short for cannabidiol, a phytocannabinoid that is found in cannabis. It is the part that can provide a lot of health benefits to animals and humans.

- Endocannabinoid: Naturally occurring cannabinoids found in the human body. When these do not work properly or there are not enough, it can take the body out of balance and make you feel unwell.

- Endocannabinoid system: The system of endocannabinoids and the enzymes that are responsible for regulating the production of endocannabinoids, and their receptors all together

.

- CB1: A cannabinoid receptor that is found mostly in the central nervous system. This includes the nerves of the spinal cord and the brain.

- CB2: Another type of cannabinoid receptor found mostly in the peripheral nervous system, the nerves that control the body outside of the spinal cord and brain.

- THC: Short for tetrahydrocannabinol. THC is a phytocannabinoid found in cannabis and can have some health benefits of animals and humans. However, this chemical is responsible for intoxicating effects that are common with marijuana use, so some people are not fond of using it.

- Entourage effect: The idea that biologically active compounds may have more biological activity when you administer them with other inactive compounds, rather than on their own.

- Hemptourage effect: The entourage effect of the compounds that are found inside of hemp-derived CBD oil and help optimize your wellness and health.

- CO2 extraction: A method used to extract the CBD from the plant. Pressurized CO_2 gas (safe, liquid form) is used to extract the oil from the plant. It has the advantage of not having a residue with the final product.

- Non-psychotoxic: The substance or chemical has no bad effects on the behavior, personality, or the mind. The user does not get high.

- Hemostasis: The self-regulating process where the body tries to find its balance.

Conclusion

Too many people suffer from ailments that diminish their quality of life. They may try various medications in search of relief. But, these medications do not always work. Even when the medications help, they often come with horrible side effects that make continuation difficult.

Many people are turning to CBD oil. Cannabis and marijuana are still misunderstood in much of the western world because of legal issues. But as the tide keeps turning, it is likely that the laws will change. When more accurate information about CBD oil comes to light, increasing numbers of individuals will look to CBD oil for help.

We have spent time considering CBD oil and how it works. We have talked about what CBD oil is, some of the legal issues surrounding it, what it can heal, how it works with your pet, and other important issues. Almost anyone can benefit from using CBD oil. It is natural and meshes well with your body's other systems.

The best way to decide if CBD is right for you is to develop a complete understanding of the product and to try it yourself. Be bold and experiment. Find out what works best for you. For many people this could well be the supplement that completely changes their lives for the better.

Thank you for taking the time to read this book. If you have gleaned valuable information from it, please take two minutes to leave a review on Amazon! It really would mean a lot to me.

Check out these other great books from the author:

Porsche 911: The Practically Free Supercar
Blockchain Basics Explained

To keep up to date with my future projects, visit me at starbunker.com or follow me on Facebook, Twitter, and Instagram.

Thank you again!

Robert McGowan

30256493R00073

Made in the USA
Lexington, KY
07 February 2019